The Thinking Tree

THE ATHLETE'S FUN-SCHOOLING JOURNAL

HOMESCHOOLING CURRICULUM HANDBOOK

FOR STUDENTS MAJORING IN SPORTS

Anna Miriam Brown &
Sarah Janisse Brown

CONTRIBUTORS:

Nancy Thomas

Samantha Carson Carver

Larinda Hessler

Amy Lynn

Kimberly Green

Meghan Nibbelin

Amanda Marie

Mindy Staley

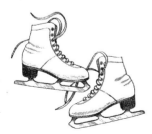

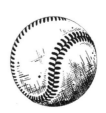

About the Athlete's Fun-Schooling Journal

This journal is designed for students majoring in sports. It's also perfect for sports fans who want to learn about different types of sports. The Sport's Fun-Schooling Journal covers traditional sports such as basketball and baseball as well as unique sports like breakdancing and kayaking. Students will even learn about chess as a sport!

To complete this guided learning journal students need books, pencils, art materials, and films/ documentaries. This journal can be used daily for an intensive sport study lasting six weeks or once a week to last the school year.

Thinking Tree Learning Levels B2, C1 & C2, ideal for ages 10+.

Topics Covered Include:

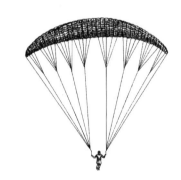

- Planning & setting priorities
- Creative writing
- Reading
- Research
- Equipment and skill study
- Film study
- News
- Nature study
- Movement and exercise
- Comics
- Math practice
- And more!

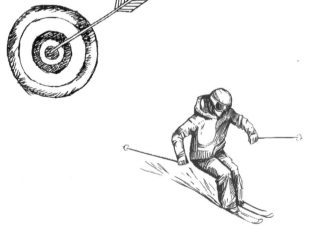

SPORTS COVERED IN THE BOOK:

Basketball	Cycling	Kayaking
Gymnastics	Boxing	Paragliding
Golf	Baseball	Rock Climbing
Hockey	Volleyball	Snowboarding
Football	Cheerleading	Swimming
Tennis	Archery	Soccer
Ping Pong	Snow Skiing	Scuba Diving
Surfing	Martial Arts	
Hiking	Hunting	And "Choose
Cricket	Figure Skating	Your Own
Breakdancing	Chess	Sport"

Instructions

Draw or list six things you want to learn about
or sports skills you want to develop:

1.

2.

3.

4.

5.

6.

Action Steps:

1. Go to the library, your bookshelf, or a bookstore.

2. Choose a total of nine books about these topics or skills.

3. Gather your supplies and get creative!

4. Complete five pages each day to develop your skills as a sports expert.

Supplies Needed:

You will need pencils, art supplies (colored
pencils or gel pens work best), and films/
documentaries. Get active! Organize your
favorite sports equipment.

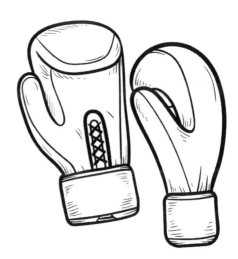

CHOOSE YOUR BOOKS

Pick out 9 different books that will help you study sports

DRAW THE COVERS AND TITLES HERE:

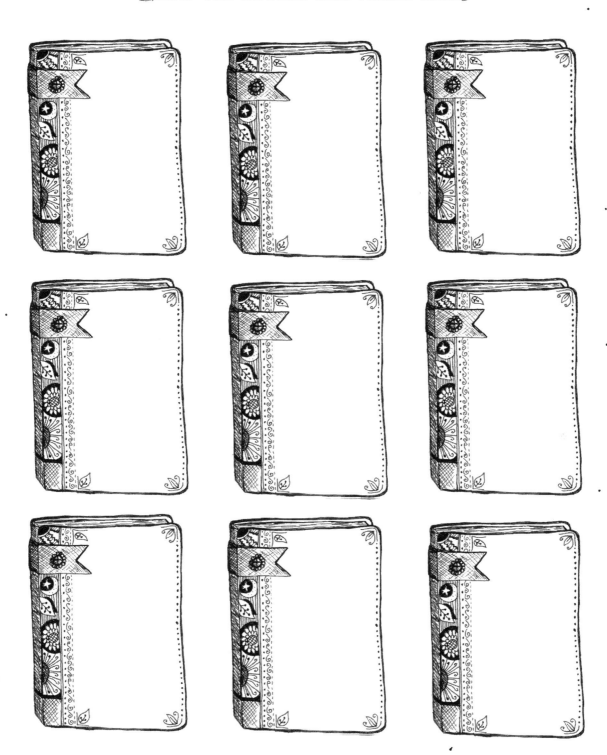

Today's Sport: Basketball

Date:_____

To-do List:

_____

_____

_____

_____

A Quote:

_____

_____

_____

_____

Today's Moods:

Today's Chores:

_____

_____

_____

_____

Books, Websites & Videos

Resources I can use to study today's sport:

_____

_____

_____

Start your day by watching a competition involving today's sport.

Math & Research Challenge

Golden State Warrior Stephen Curry's 2018-2019 stats show the percentage of three-point shots he made was 43.7%. If he attempted 810 shots, how many did he make?

Solve the challenge:

_____
_____
_____
_____
_____
_____

ANSWER:

_____

Illustrate your answer:

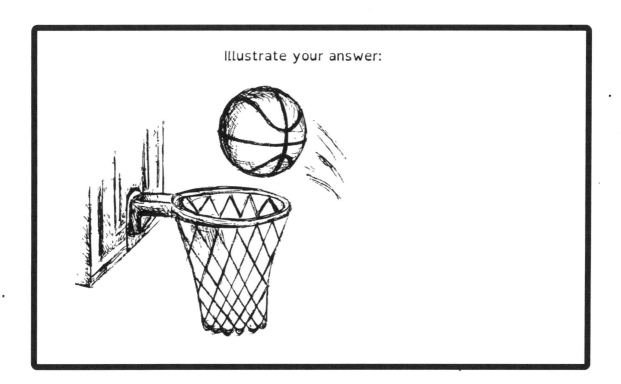

Sports Study

Basketball

It's research time!

Use the Internet, books, tutorials and documentaries to study this sport. Or go see a game or competition!

Draw any equipment needed for this sport.

Draw a player in uniform.

Draw a trophy or medal for this sport.

Where did this sport originate from?

_____

_____

How was this sport invented?

_____

_____

_____

Who are the main sponsors of the events for this sport?

_____

_____

What is the name of the largest competition where this sport is played? _____

_____

_____

_____

Who is the #1 player of this sport? What makes them the best? How much money do they earn? Where do their earnings come from?

_____

_____

_____

_____

Would you like to play this sport? Why or why not?

_____

_____

What are the common injuries from playing this sport?

_____

_____

_____

Random fact about this sport.

_____

_____

_____

Say What?

Invent your own comic book font and add words to the picture

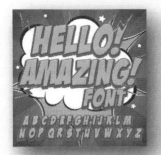
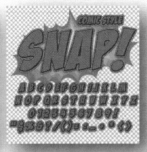
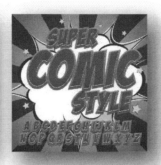
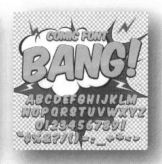

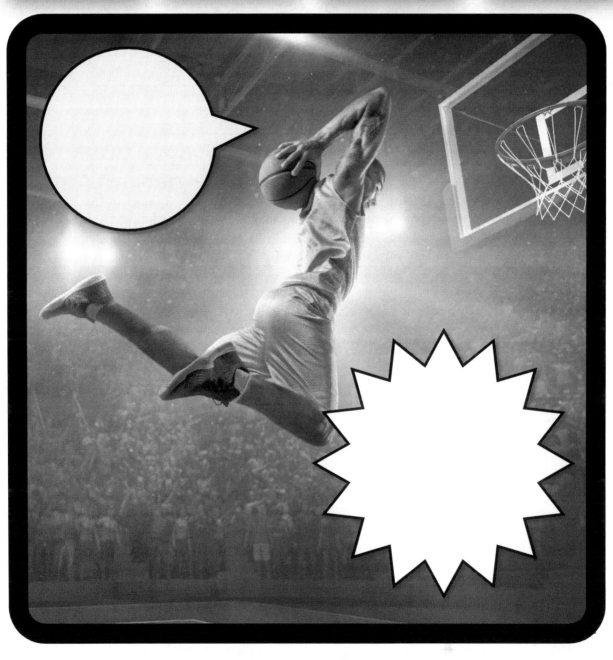

Sports News

Open a newspaper or look online!

What is happening in the world of sports today?

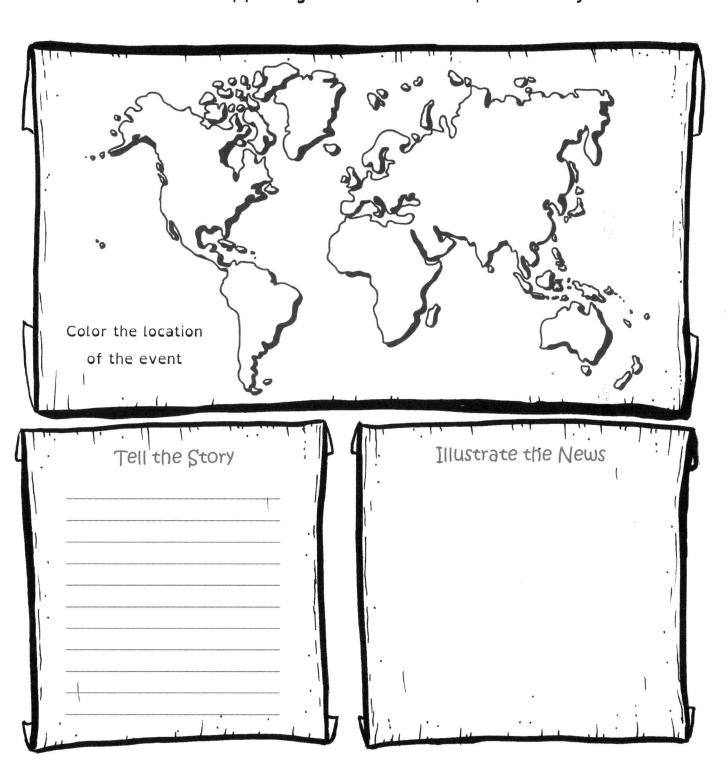

Color the location
of the event

Tell the Story

Illustrate the News

Screen Time

Watch a high-quality film, video, tutorial or sports documentary.

Title_____

Screen Time_____

Producer_____

Actors_____

_____

_____

_____

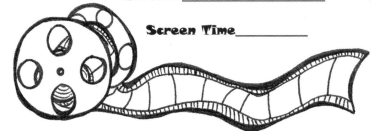

Quotes

Draw a scene from the video.

Rating:

worst

Bad

Awful

Ok

Nice

Great

Best

Make a Comic

From the video or your imagination.

Title_____

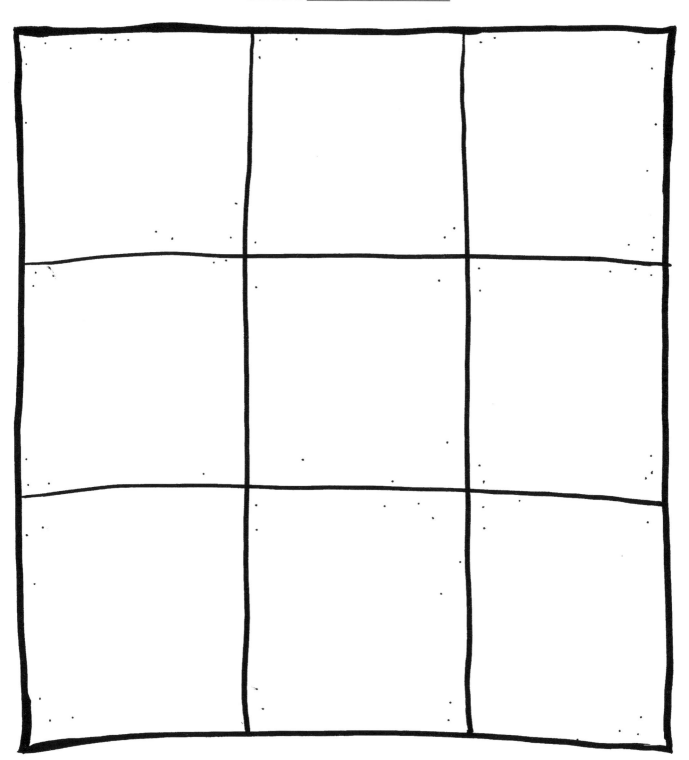

Drawing & Reading Time!

Choose a few books from your stack to focus on today.

Write down and draw anything that inspires you.

(Set a timer for 1 hour)

Free time!

Set the timer for 30 minutes and go outside to play,
explore and practice a sport.

What do you plan to do on your free time?

What do you want to practice?

Do you have any goals?

Draw your goals!

Math Practice

Use this page for math practice,

or design a sport's field, rink or play zone

for the sport you are studying today!

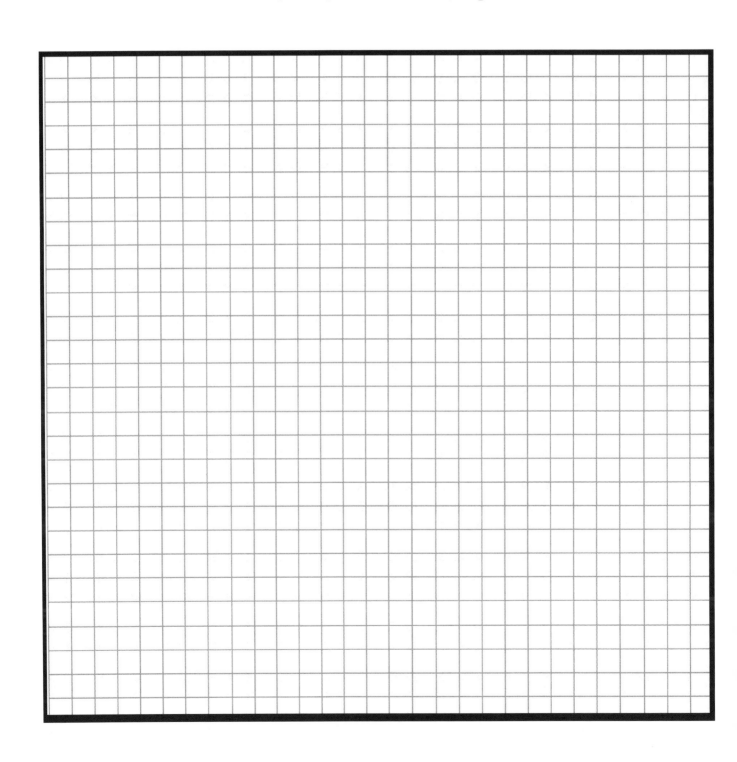

Nature Study

Take this book outside and draw anything and everything that inspires you.

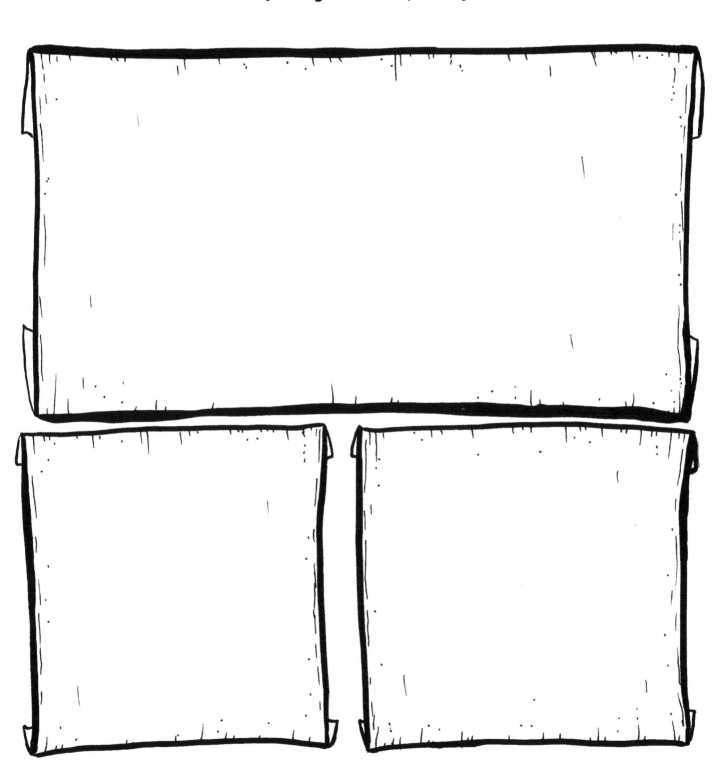

Today's Sport: Gymnastics

Date:_____

To-do List:

_____
_____
_____
_____

A Quote:

_____
_____
_____
_____

Today's Moods:

Today's Chores:

_____
_____
_____
_____

Books, Websites & Videos

Resources I can use to study today's sport:

_____
_____
_____

Start your day by watching a competition involving today's sport.

Math & Research Challenge

Maggie needs at least a 32.5 overall score to make state. Her floor routine scored a 9.2, but her beam routine was only an 8.1; What does she need to average on bars and vault to make state?

Solve the challenge:

_____
_____
_____
_____
_____
_____

ANSWER:

_____

Illustrate your answer:

Sports Study

Gymnastics

It's research time!

Use the Internet, books, tutorials and documentaries to study this sport. Or go see a game or competition!

Draw any equipment needed for this sport.

Draw a player in uniform.

Draw a trophy or medal for this sport.

Where did this sport originate from?

_____

_____

How was this sport invented?

_____

_____

_____

Who are the main sponsors of the events for this sport?

_____

_____

What is the name of the largest competition where this sport is played? _____

_____

_____

_____

_____

Who is the #1 player of this sport? What makes them the best? How much money do they earn? Where do their earnings come from?

_____

_____

_____

_____

_____

Would you like to play this sport? Why or why not?

_____

_____

_____

What are the common injuries from playing this sport?

_____

_____

_____

_____

Random fact about this sport.

_____

_____

_____

Say What?

Invent your own comic book font and add words to the picture

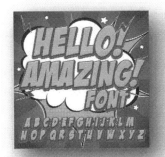
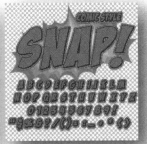
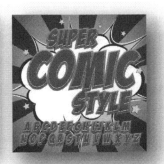
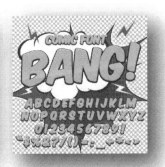

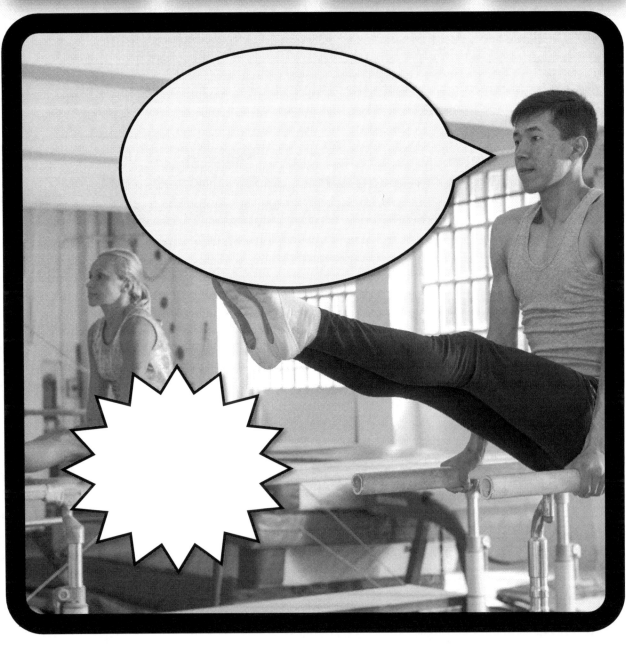

Sports News

Open a newspaper or look online!

What is happening in the world of sports today?

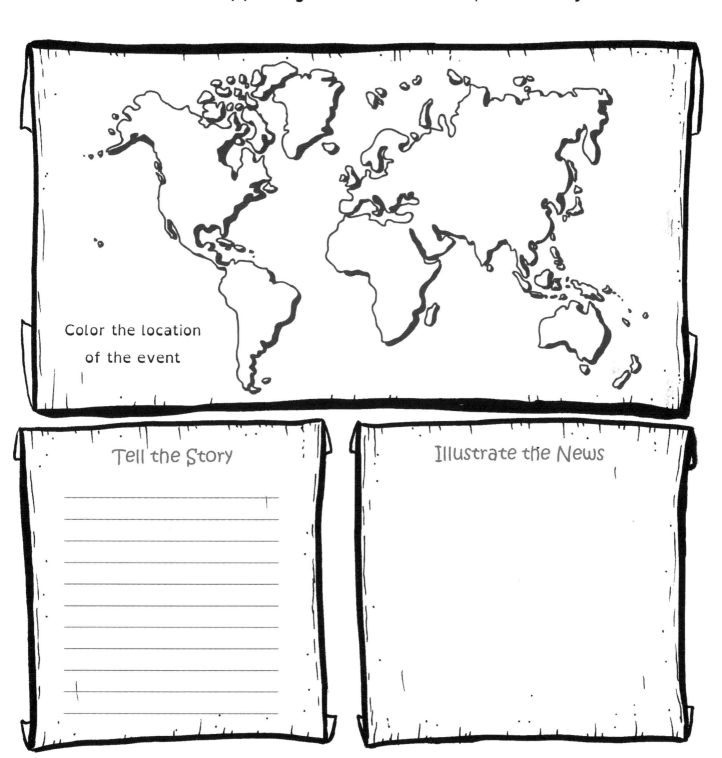

Color the location
of the event

Tell the Story

Illustrate the News

Screen Time

Watch a high-quality film, video, tutorial or sports documentary.

Title_____

Screen Time_____

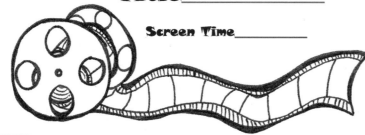

Producer_____

Actors_____

_____

_____

_____

Quotes

Draw a scene from the video.

Rating:

worst

Bad

Awful

Ok

Nice

Great

Best

Make a Comic

From the video or your imagination.

Title_____

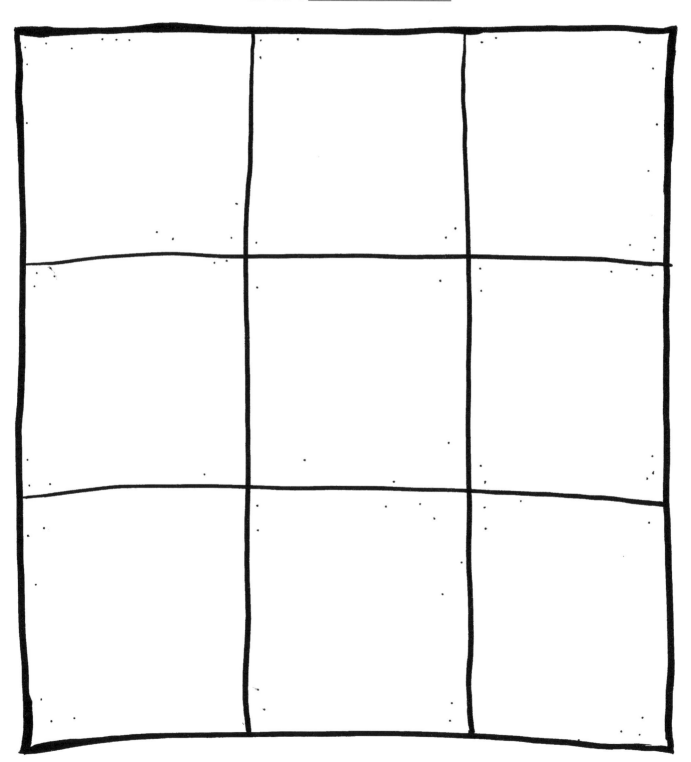

Drawing & Reading Time!

Choose a few books from your stack to focus on today.

Write down and draw anything that inspires you.

(Set a timer for 1 hour)

Free time!

Set the timer for 30 minutes and go outside to play, explore and practice a sport.

What do you plan to do on your free time?

_____

_____

What do you want to practice?

_____

_____

Do you have any goals?

_____

_____

Draw your goals!

Math Practice

Use this page for math practice,

or design a sport's field, rink or play zone

for the sport you are studying today!

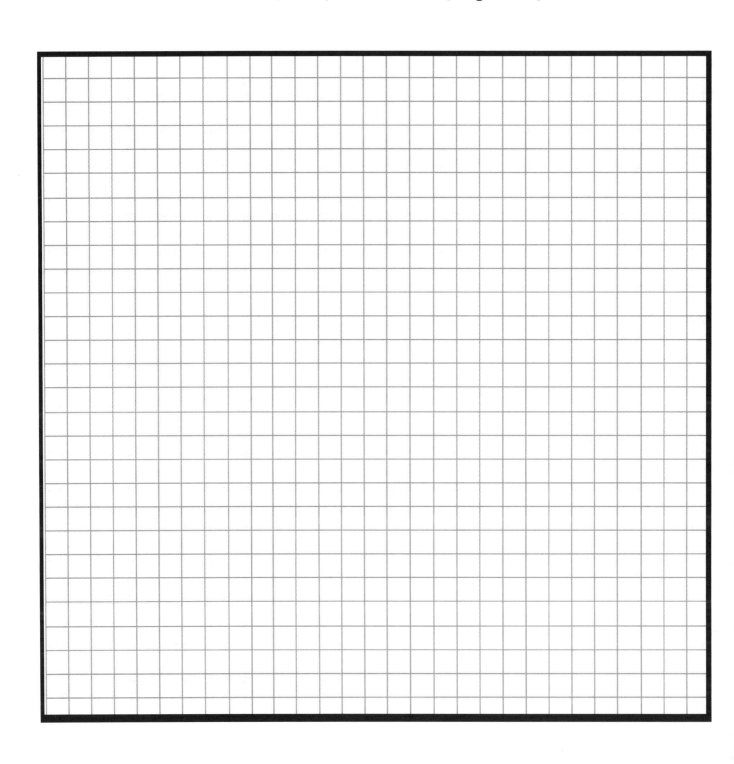

Nature Study

Take this book outside and draw anything and
everything that inspires you.

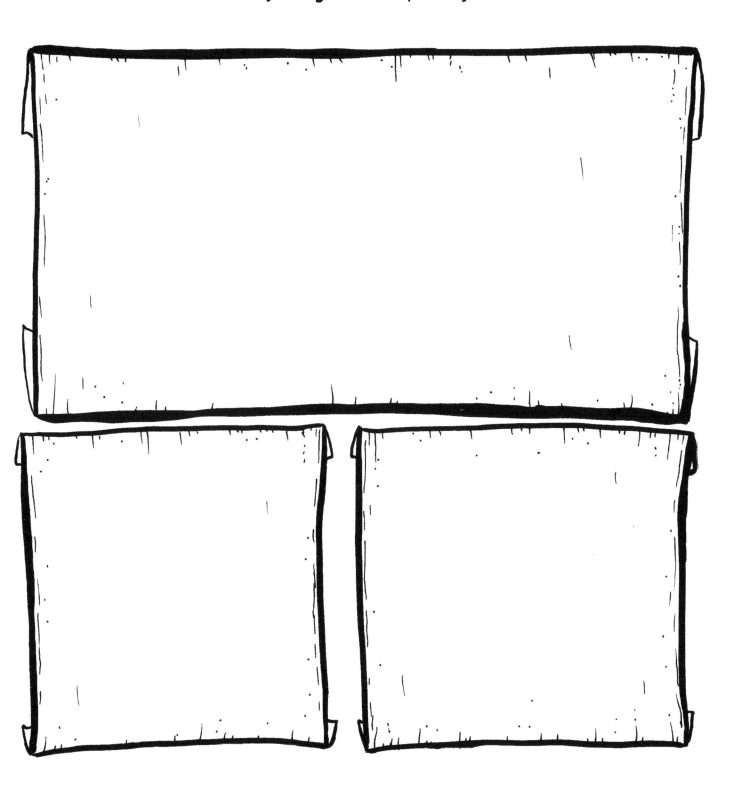

Today's Sport: Golf

Date:_____

To-do List:
_____
_____
_____
_____

A Quote:
_____
_____
_____
_____

Today's Moods:

Today's Chores:
_____
_____
_____
_____

Books, Websites & Videos

Resources I can use to study today's sport:

_____
_____
_____

Start your day by watching a competition involving today's sport.

Math & Research Challenge

Jaylin swings her club at 5 different golf balls. She hits 2 of the balls. What fraction of balls did she hit? What fraction did she miss? If she hit 2 times as many balls, what fraction of balls would she have hit?

Solve the challenge:

_____
_____
_____
_____
_____
_____

ANSWER:

_____

Illustrate your answer:

Sports Study

Golf

It's research time!

Use the Internet, books, tutorials and documentaries to study
this sport. Or go see a game or competition!

Draw any equipment needed for this sport.

Draw a player in uniform.

Draw a trophy or medal for this sport.

Where did this sport originate from?

_____

_____

How was this sport invented?

_____

_____

_____

Who are the main sponsors of the events for this sport?

_____

_____

What is the name of the largest competition where this sport is played? _____

_____

_____

_____

_____

Who is the #1 player of this sport? What makes them the best? How much money do they earn? Where do their earnings come from?

_____

_____

_____

_____

Would you like to play this sport? Why or why not?

_____

_____

What are the common injuries from playing this sport?

_____

_____

_____

Random fact about this sport.

_____

_____

_____

Say What?

Invent your own comic book font and add words to the picture

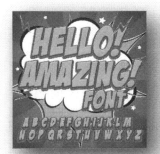
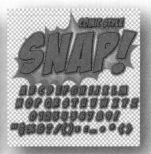
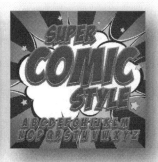
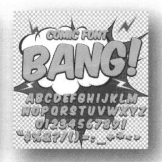

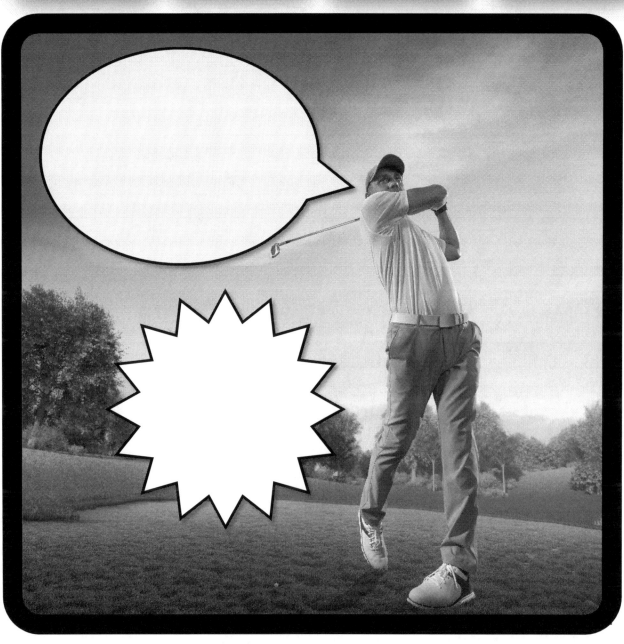

Sports News

Open a newspaper or look online!

What is happening in the world of sports today?

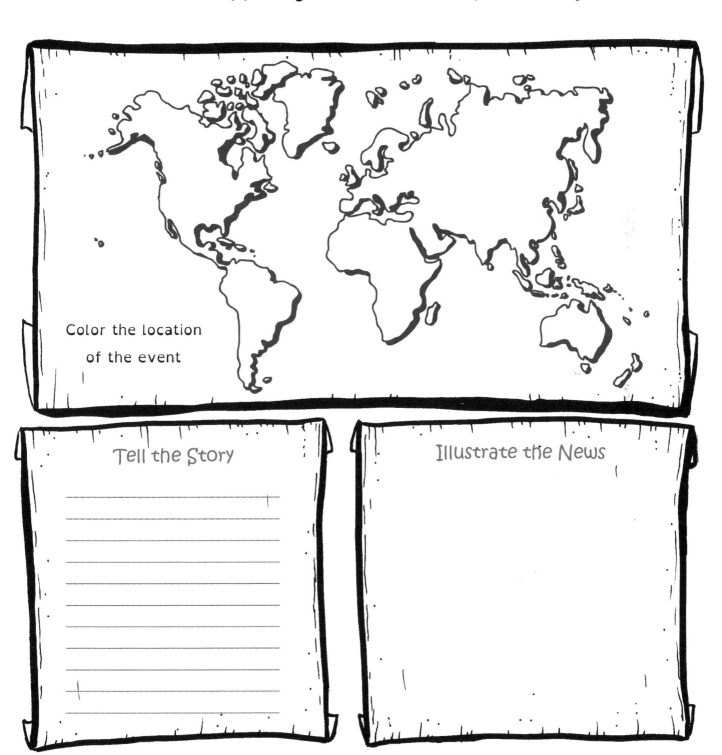

Color the location
of the event

Tell the Story

Illustrate the News

Screen Time

Watch a high-quality film, video, tutorial or sports documentary.

Title_____

Screen Time_____

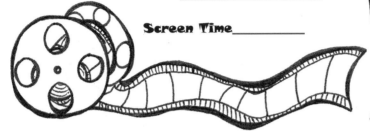

Producer_____

Actors_____

_____

_____

_____

Quotes

Draw a scene from the video.

Rating:

worst

Bad

Awful

Ok

Nice

Great

Best

Make a Comic

From the video or your imagination.

Title_____

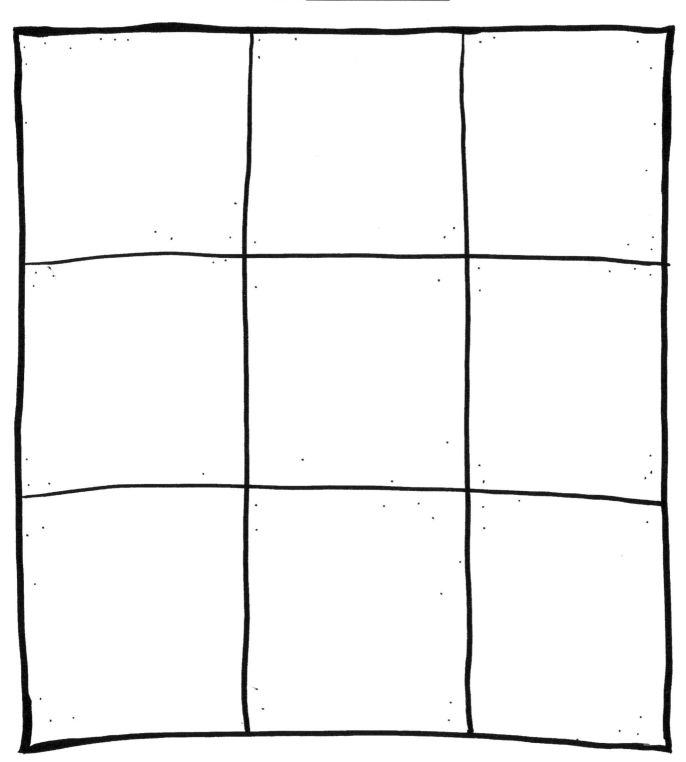

Drawing & Reading Time!

Choose a few books from your stack to focus on today.

Write down and draw anything that inspires you.

(Set a timer for 1 hour)

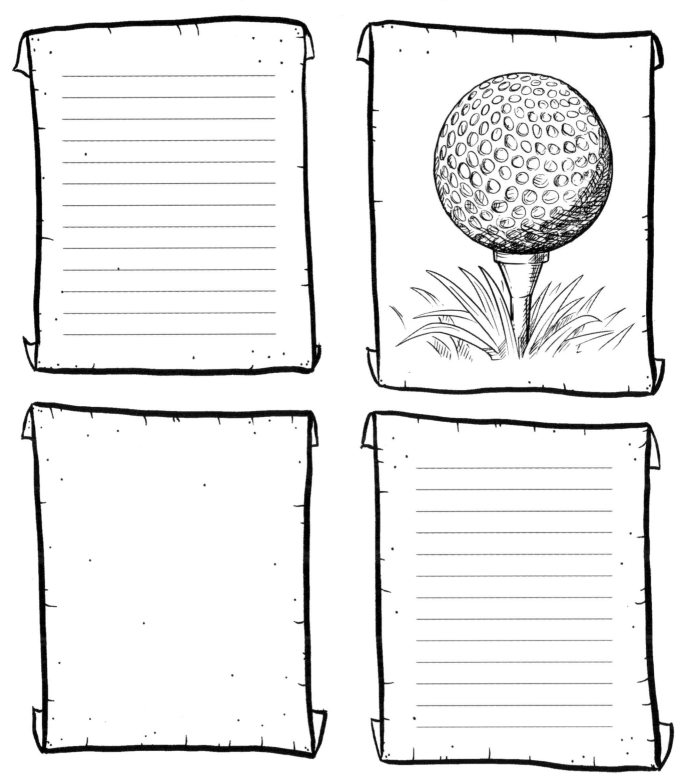

Free time!

Set the timer for 30 minutes and go outside to play, explore and practice a sport.

What do you plan to do on your free time?

_____

_____

What do you want to practice?

_____

_____

Do you have any goals?

_____

_____

Draw your goals!

Math Practice

Use this page for math practice,

or design a sport's field, rink or play zone

for the sport you are studying today!

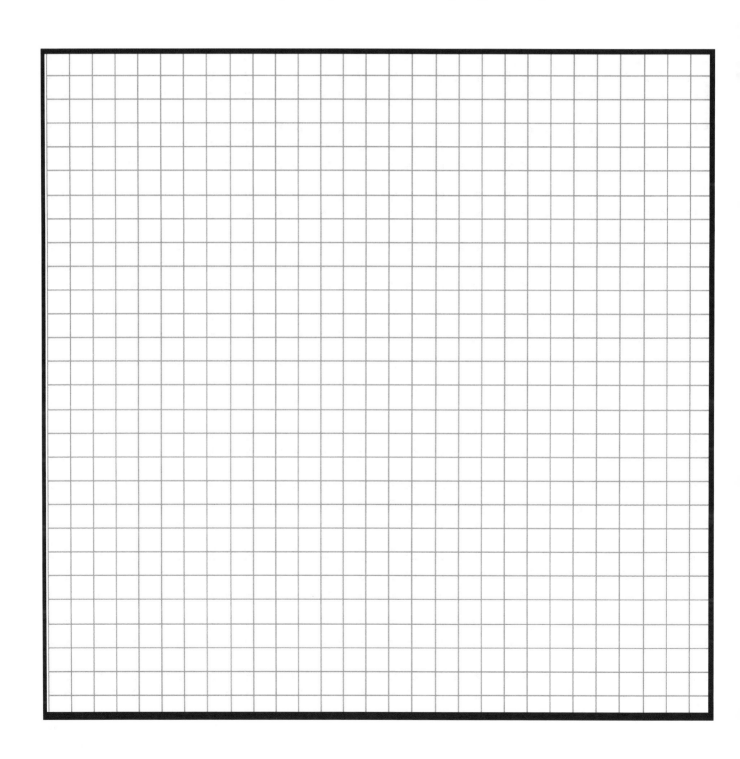

Nature Study

Take this book outside and draw anything and everything that inspires you.

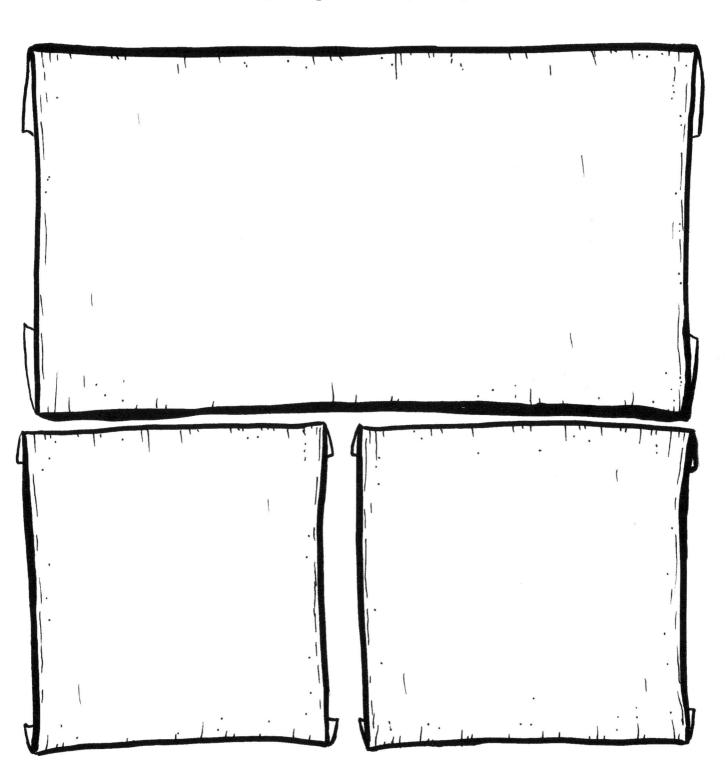

Today's Sport: Hockey

Date:_____

To-do List:
_____
_____
_____
_____

A Quote:
_____
_____
_____
_____

Today's Moods:

Today's Chores:
_____
_____
_____
_____

Books, Websites & Videos

Resources I can use to study today's sport:

_____
_____
_____

Start your day by watching a competition involving today's sport.

Math & Research Challenge

Hockey is played on ice. What state of matter is ice: liquid, gas, or solid? At what temperature does water freeze? What atoms make up ice? What temperature does water have to be at to turn into a gas?

Solve the challenge:

_____
_____
_____
_____
_____
_____

ANSWER:

_____

Illustrate your answer:

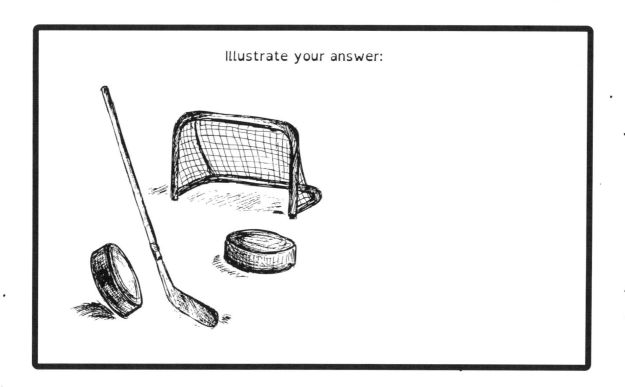

Sports Study

Hockey

It's research time!

Use the Internet, books, tutorials and documentaries to study this sport. Or go see a game or competition!

Draw any equipment needed for this sport.

Draw a player in uniform.

Draw a trophy or medal for this sport.

Where did this sport originate from?

_____

_____

How was this sport invented?

_____

_____

_____

Who are the main sponsors of the events for this sport?

_____

_____

What is the name of the largest competition where this sport is played? _____

_____

_____

_____

_____

Who is the #1 player of this sport? What makes them the best? How much money do they earn? Where do their earnings come from?

_____

_____

_____

_____

Would you like to play this sport? Why or why not?

_____

_____

What are the common injuries from playing this sport?

_____

_____

_____

Random fact about this sport.

_____

_____

_____

Say What?

Invent your own comic book font and add words to the picture

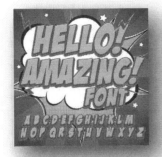
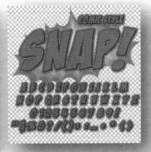
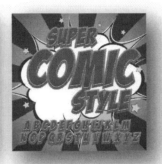
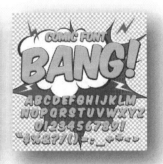

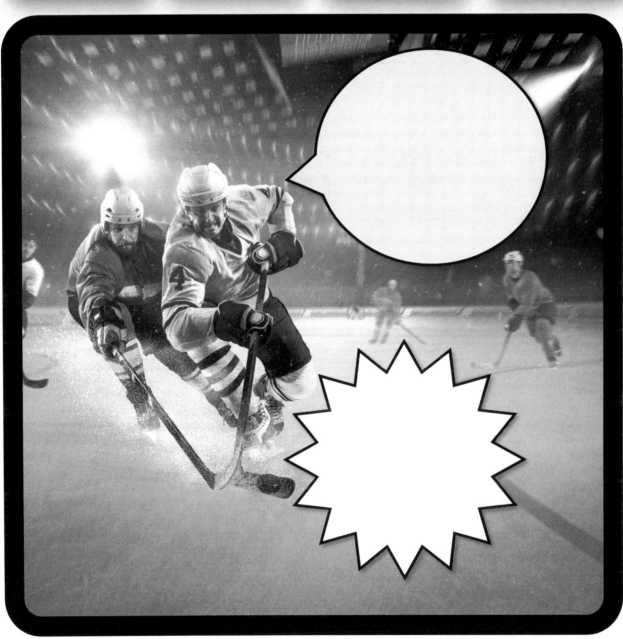

Sports News

Open a newspaper or look online!

What is happening in the world of sports today?

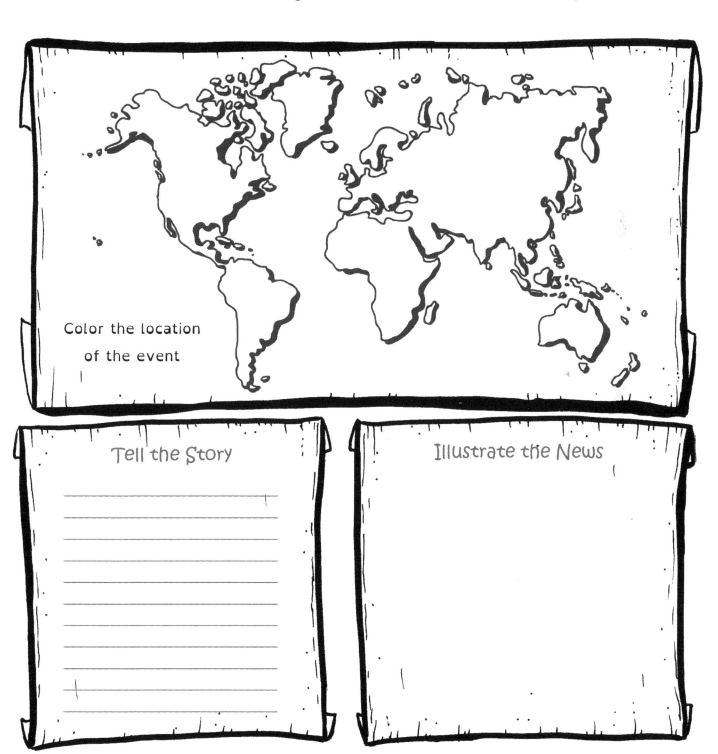

Color the location
of the event

Tell the Story

Illustrate the News

Screen Time

Watch a high-quality film, video, tutorial or sports documentary.

Title_____

Screen Time_____

Producer_____

Actors_____

_____

_____

_____

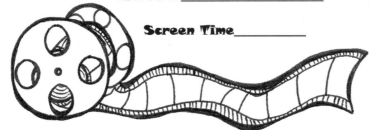

Quotes

Draw a scene from the video.

Rating:

worst

Bad

Awful

Ok

Nice

Great

Best

Make a Comic

From the video or your imagination.

Title_____

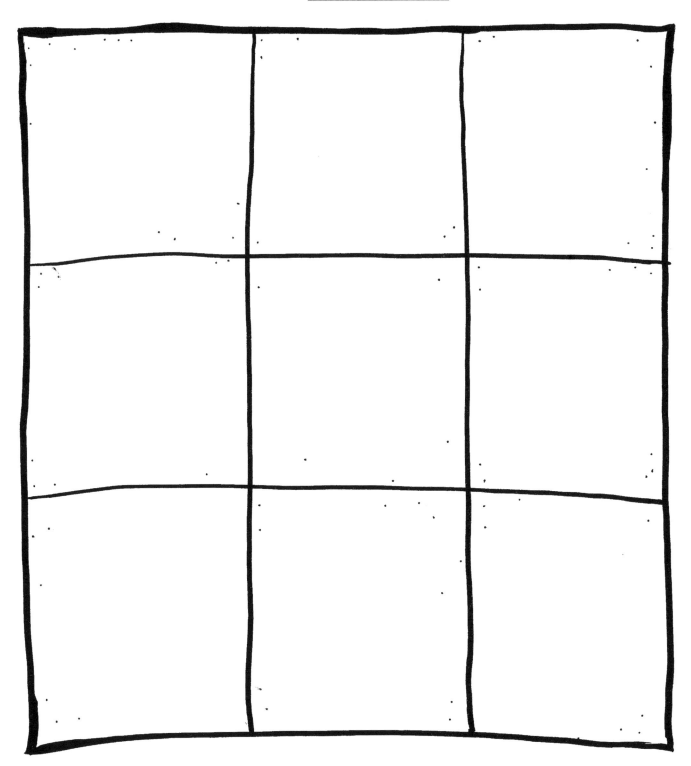

Drawing & Reading Time!

Choose a few books from your stack to focus on today.

Write down and draw anything that inspires you.

(Set a timer for 1 hour)

Free time!

Set the timer for 30 minutes and go outside to play, explore and practice a sport.

What do you plan to do on your free time?

_____

_____

What do you want to practice?

_____

_____

Do you have any goals?

_____

_____

Draw your goals!

Math Practice

Use this page for math practice,

or design a sport's field, rink or play zone

for the sport you are studying today!

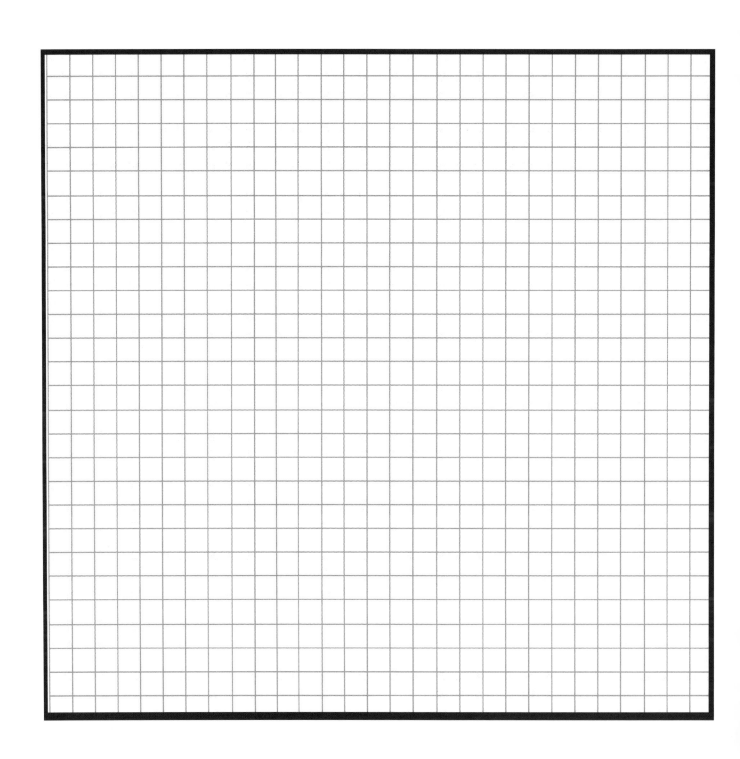

Nature Study

Take this book outside and draw anything and everything that inspires you.

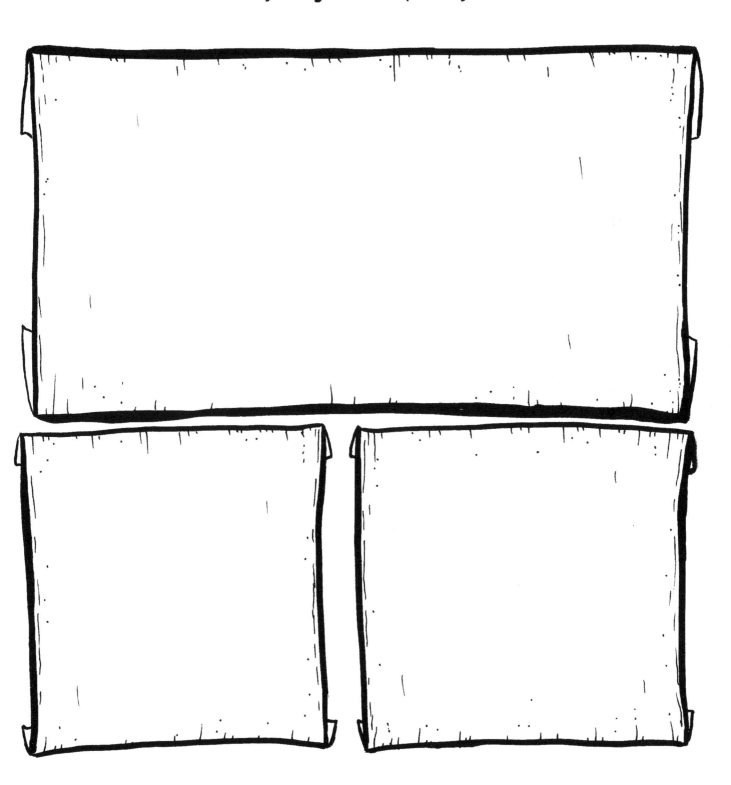

Today's Sport: Football

Date:_____

To-do List:
_____
_____
_____
_____

A Quote:
_____
_____
_____
_____

Today's Moods:

Today's Chores:
_____
_____
_____
_____

Books, Websites & Videos

Resources I can use to study today's sport:

_____
_____
_____

Start your day by watching a competition involving today's sport.

Math & Research Challenge

A touchdown is worth 7 points, and a field goal is worth 3 points. The Cowboys scored 5 touchdowns and 2 field goals. The Packers scored 6 touchdowns and 1 field goal. What was the final score? Who won?

Solve the challenge:

_____

_____

_____

_____

_____

_____

ANSWER:

_____

Illustrate your answer:

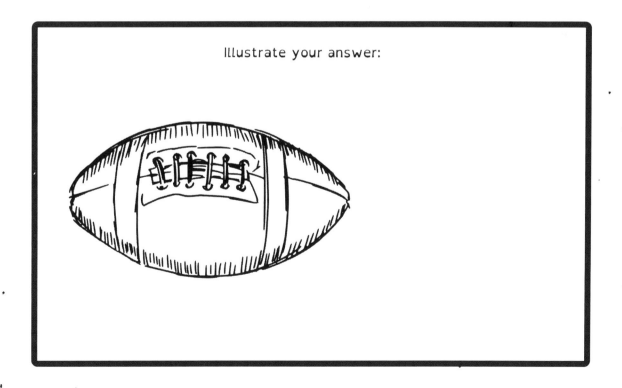

Sports Study

Football

It's research time!

Use the Internet, books, tutorials and documentaries to study this sport. Or go see a game or competition!

Draw any equipment needed for this sport.

Draw a player in uniform.

Draw a trophy or medal for this sport.

Where did this sport originate from?

_____

_____

How was this sport invented?

_____

_____

_____

Who are the main sponsors of the events for this sport?

_____

_____

What is the name of the largest competition where this sport is played? _____

_____

_____

_____

_____

Who is the #1 player of this sport? What makes them the best? How much money do they earn? Where do their earnings come from?

_____

_____

_____

_____

_____

Would you like to play this sport? Why or why not?

_____

_____

_____

What are the common injuries from playing this sport?

_____

_____

_____

_____

Random fact about this sport.

_____

_____

_____

Say What?

Invent your own comic book font and add words to the picture

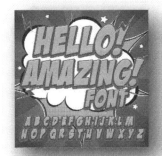
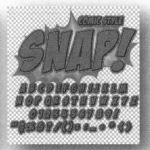
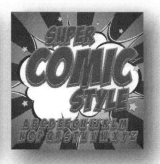
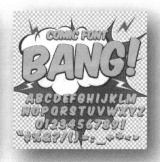

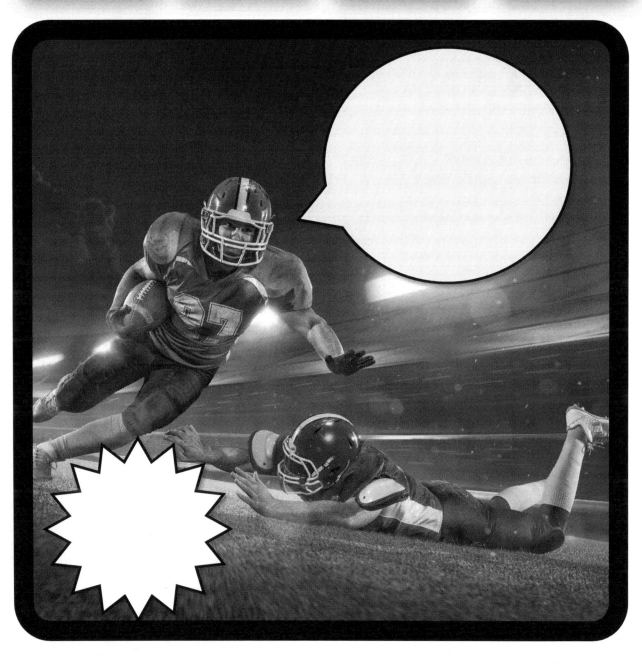

Sports News

Open a newspaper or look online!

What is happening in the world of sports today?

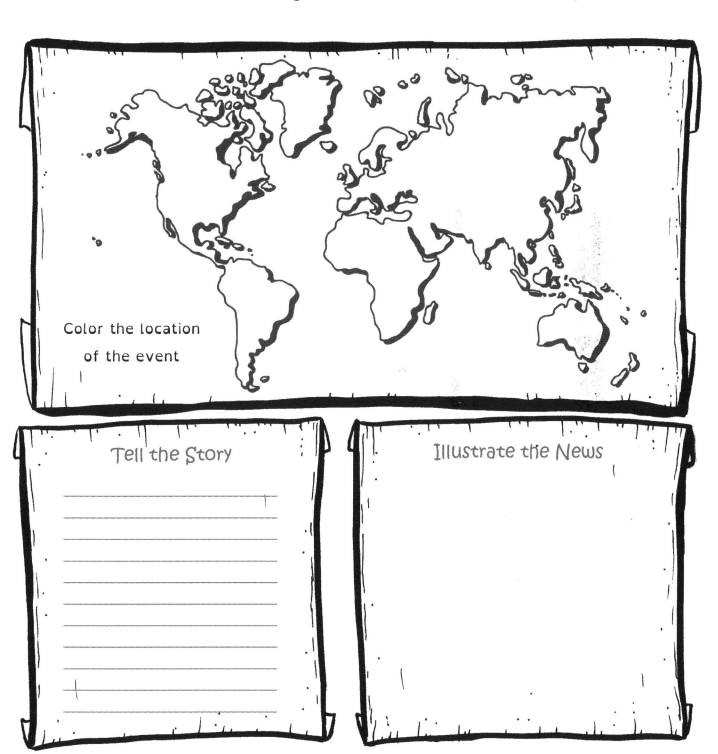

Color the location
of the event

Tell the Story

Illustrate the News

Screen Time

Watch a high-quality film, video, tutorial or sports documentary.

Title_____

Screen Time_____

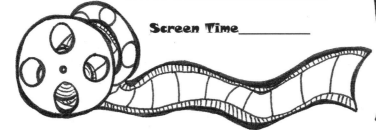

Producer_____

Actors_____

_____

_____

_____

Quotes

Draw a scene from the video.

Rating:

worst

Bad

Awful

Ok

Nice

Great

Best

Make a Comic

From the video or your imagination.

Title_____

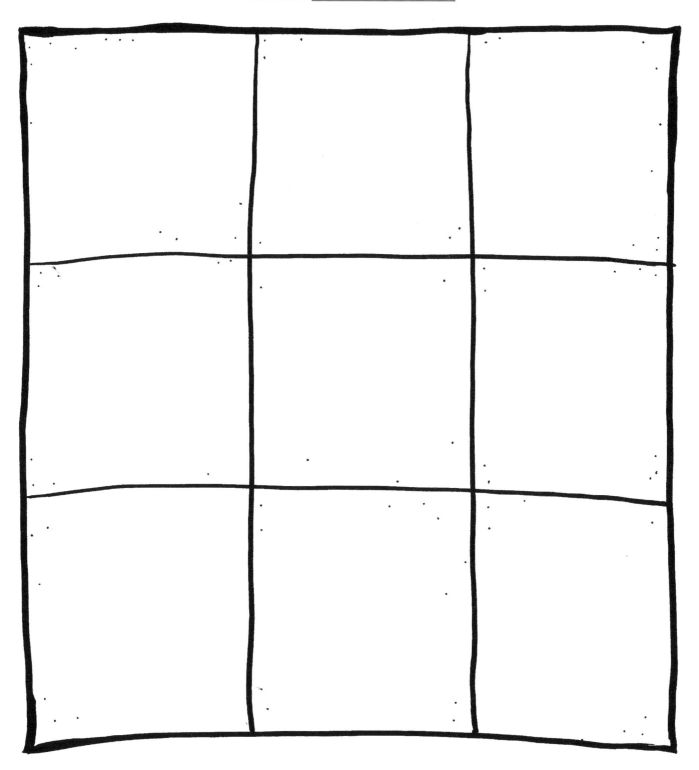

Drawing & Reading Time!

Choose a few books from your stack to focus on today.

Write down and draw anything that inspires you.

(Set a timer for 1 hour)

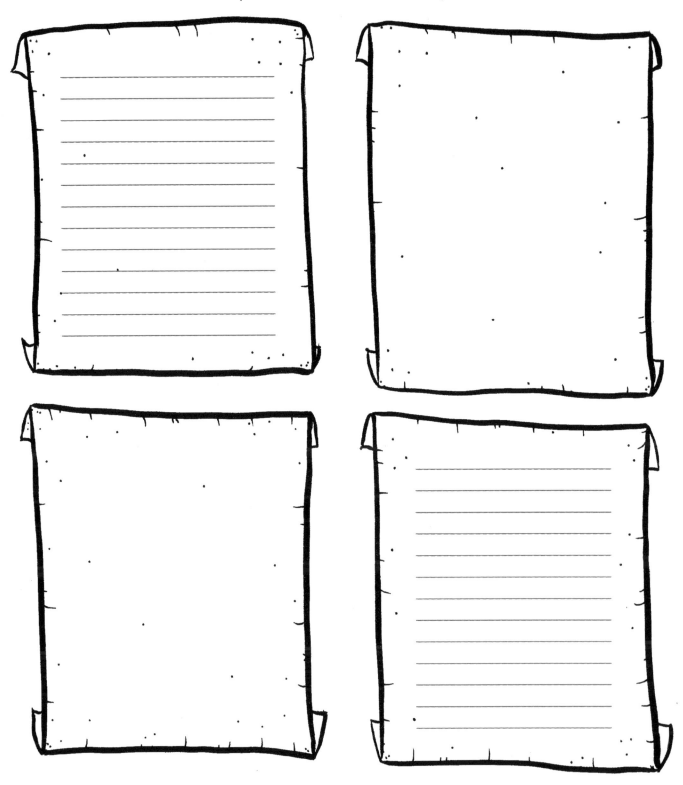

Free time!

Set the timer for 30 minutes and go outside to play, explore and practice a sport.

What do you plan to do on your free time?

What do you want to practice?

Do you have any goals?

Draw your goals!

Math Practice

Use this page for math practice,
or design a sport's field, rink or play zone
for the sport you are studying today!

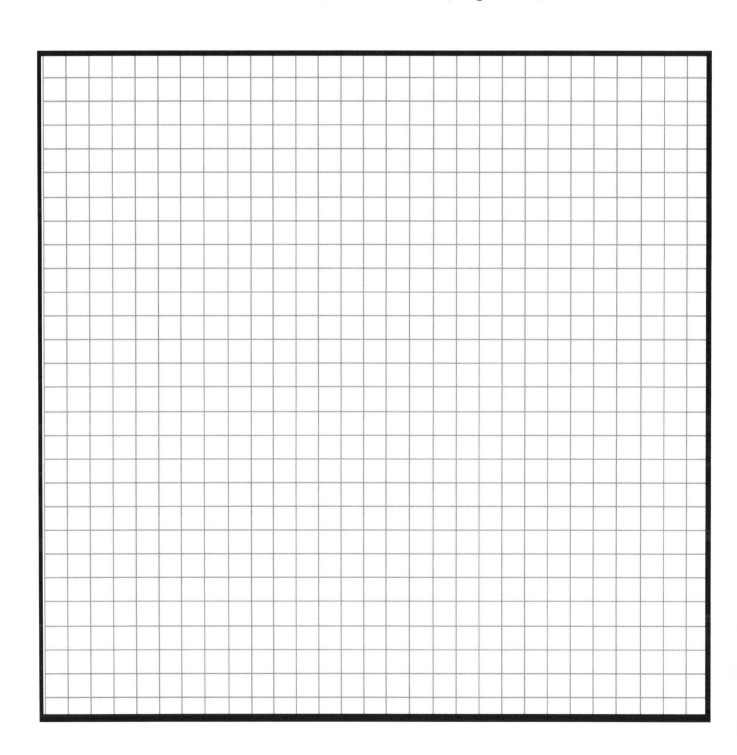

Nature Study

Take this book outside and draw anything and everything that inspires you.

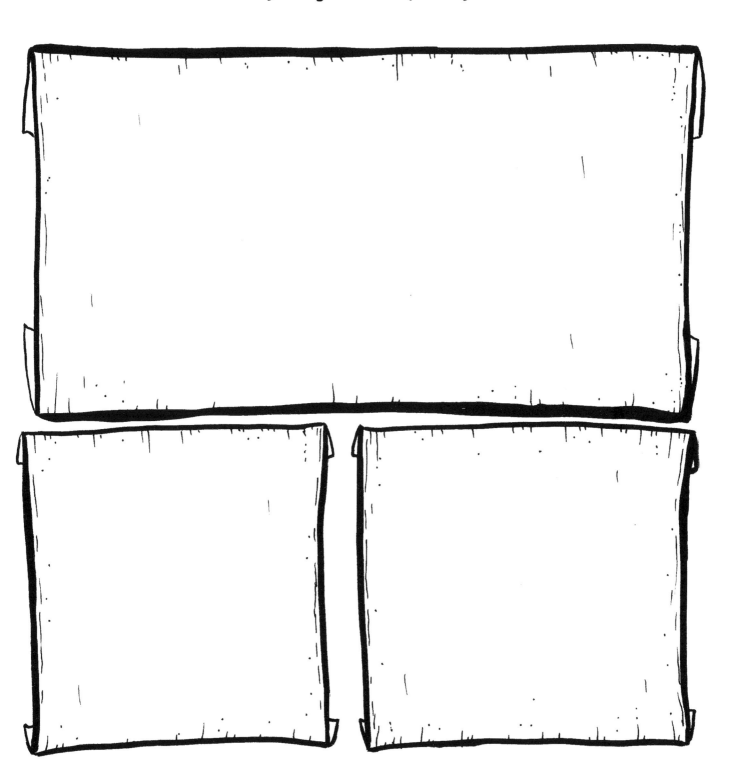

Today's Sport: Tennis

Date:_____

To-do List:

_____
_____
_____
_____
_____

A Quote:

_____
_____
_____
_____
_____

Today's Moods:

Today's Chores:

_____
_____
_____
_____

Books, Websites & Videos

Resources I can use to study today's sport:

_____
_____
_____

Start your day by watching a competition involving today's sport.

Finish the Story

The set was all tied up at 6 games each, and the tie breaker would determine the winner of the first set. Eden prepared to receive the serve. Hope tossed the tennis ball in the air and followed through with a powerful swing, just as a golden yellow dog sprinted onto the court...

_____

_____

_____

_____

_____

_____

_____

Illustrate your story:

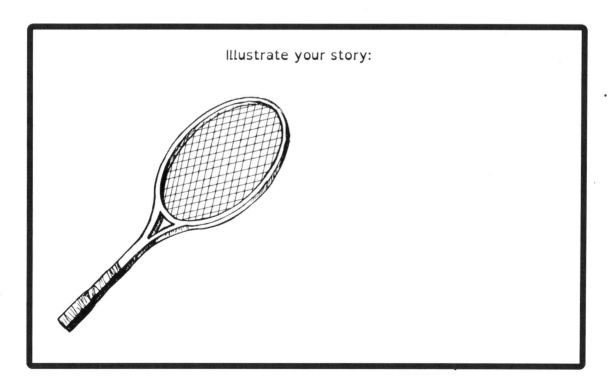

Sports Study

Tennis

It's research time!

Use the Internet, books, tutorials and documentaries to study
this sport. Or go see a game or competition!

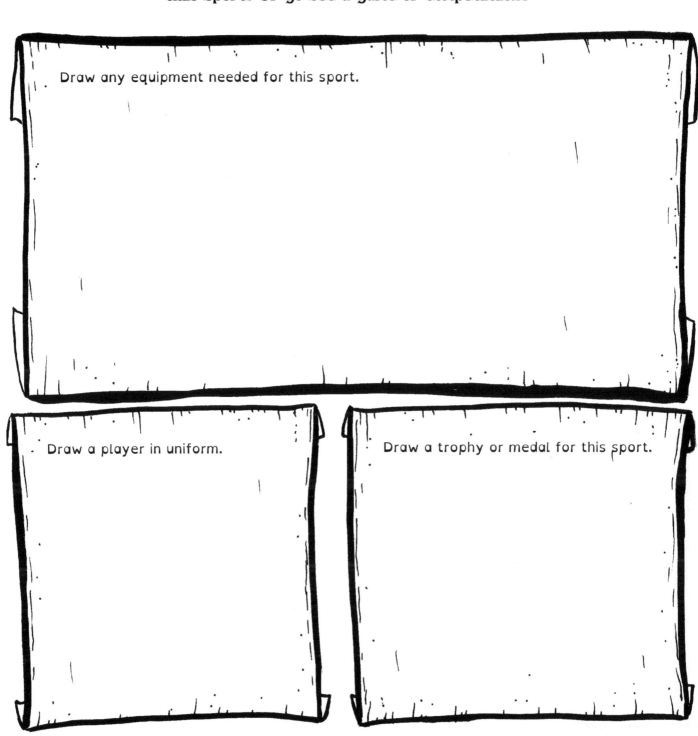

Draw any equipment needed for this sport.

Draw a player in uniform.

Draw a trophy or medal for this sport.

Where did this sport originate from?

_____

_____

How was this sport invented?

_____

_____

_____

Who are the main sponsors of the events for this sport?

_____

_____

What is the name of the largest competition where this sport is played? _____

_____

_____

_____

Who is the #1 player of this sport? What makes them the best? How much money do they earn? Where do their earnings come from?

_____

_____

_____

_____

Would you like to play this sport? Why or why not?

_____

_____

What are the common injuries from playing this sport?

_____

_____

_____

Random fact about this sport.

_____

_____

_____

Say What?

Invent your own comic book font and add words to the picture

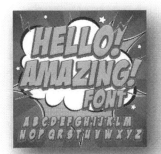 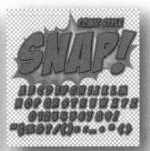 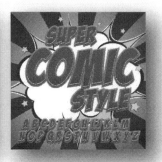 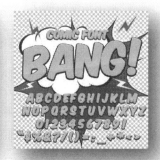

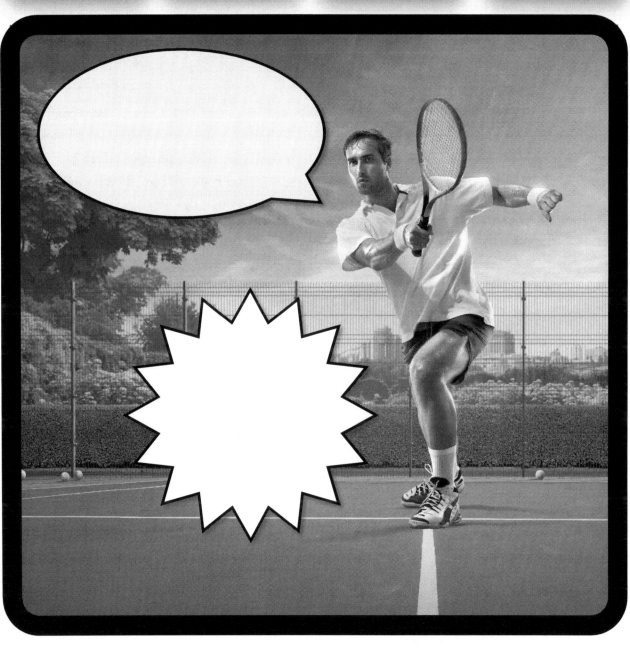

Sports News

Open a newspaper or look online!

What is happening in the world of sports today?

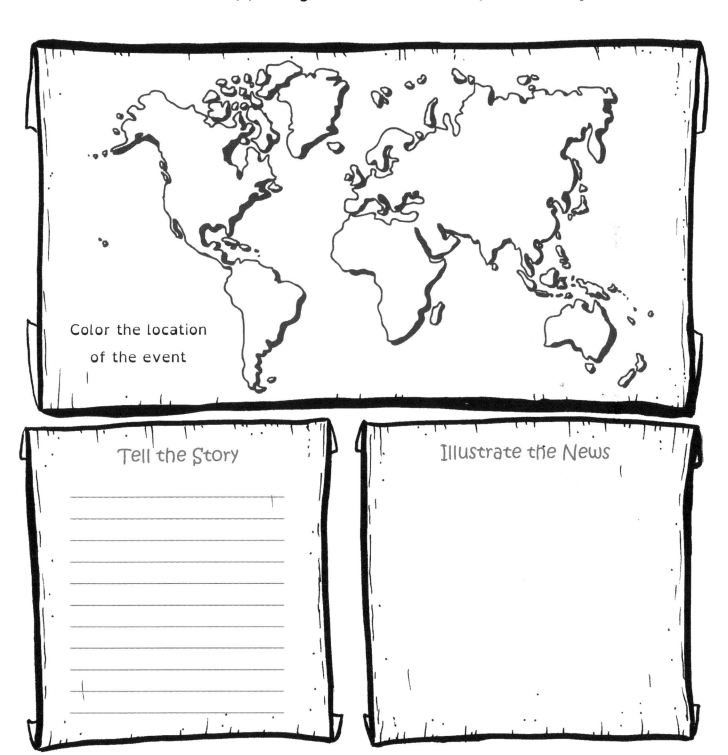

Color the location of the event

Tell the Story

Illustrate the News

Screen Time

Watch a high-quality film, video, tutorial or sports documentary.

Title_____

Screen Time_____

Producer_____

Actors_____

_____

_____

_____

Quotes

Draw a scene from the video.

Rating:

worst

Bad

Awful

Ok

Nice

Great

Best

Make a Comic

From the video or your imagination.

Title_____

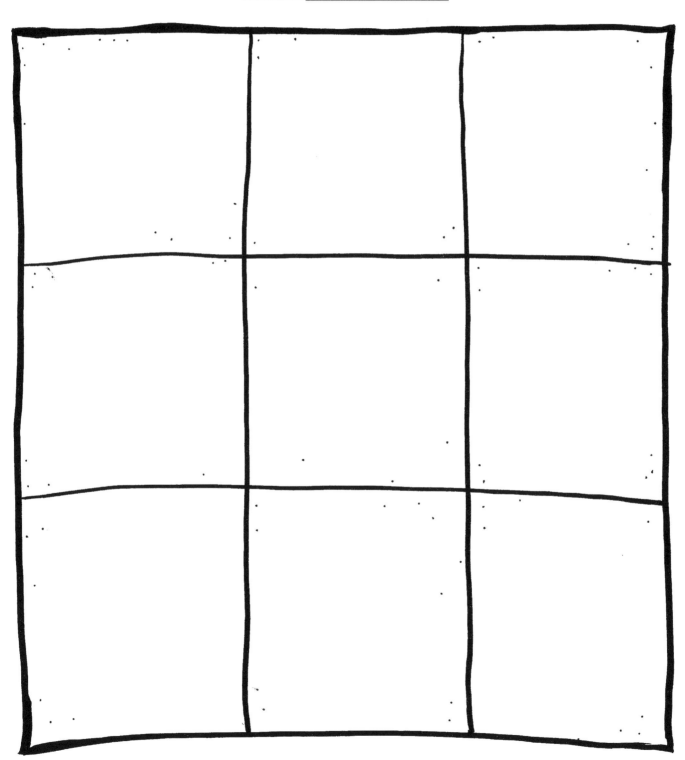

Drawing & Reading Time!

Choose a few books from your stack to focus on today.

Write down and draw anything that inspires you.

(Set a timer for 1 hour)

Free time!

Set the timer for 30 minutes and go outside to play, explore and practice a sport.

What do you plan to do on your free time?

_____

_____

What do you want to practice?

_____

_____

Do you have any goals?

_____

_____

Draw your goals!

Math Practice

Use this page for math practice,
or design a sport's field, rink or play zone
for the sport you are studying today!

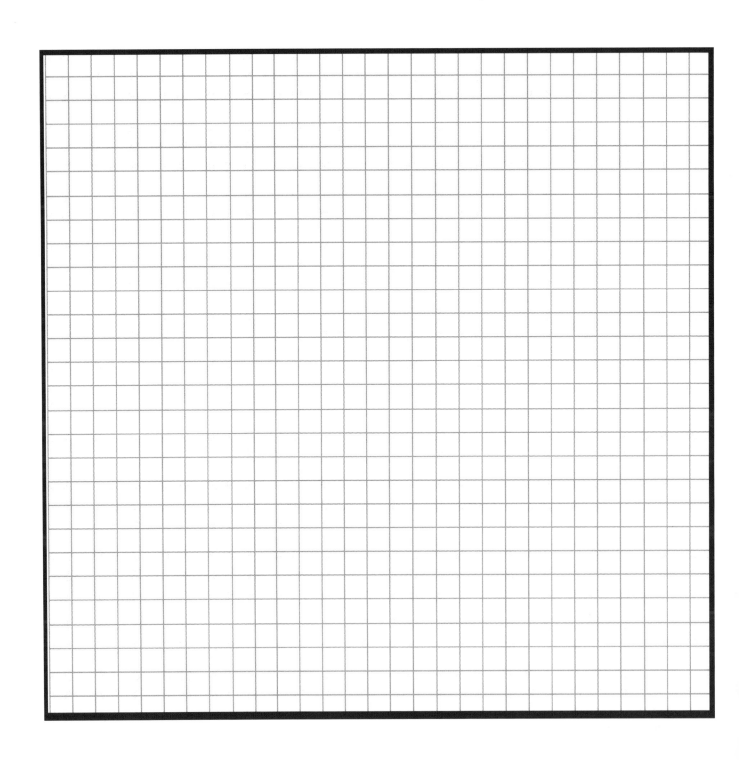

Nature Study

Take this book outside and draw anything and everything that inspires you.

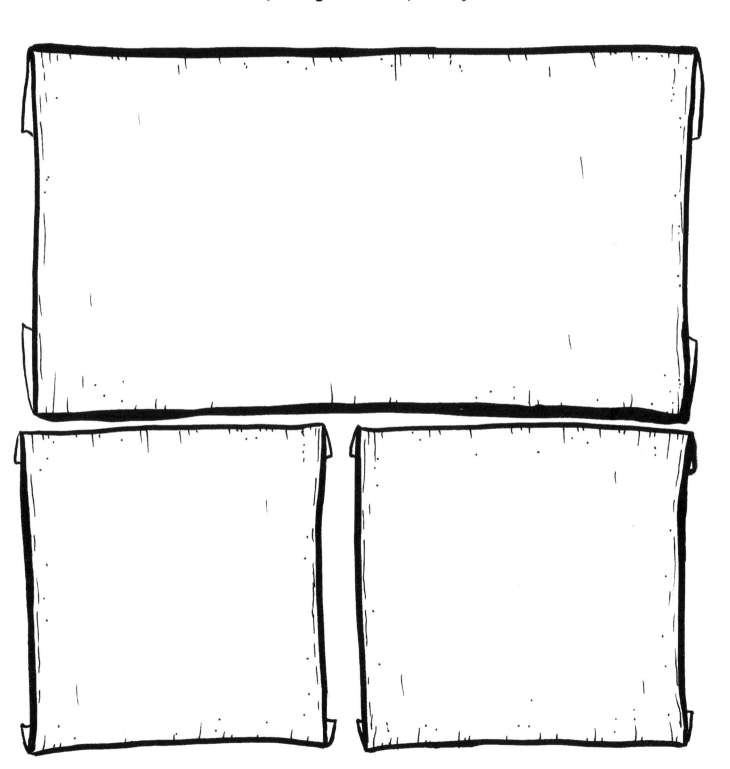

Today's Sport: Ping Pong

Date:_____

To-do List:

_____
_____
_____
_____
_____

A Quote:

_____
_____
_____
_____
_____

Today's Moods:

Today's Chores:

_____
_____
_____
_____

Books, Websites & Videos

Resources I can use to study today's sport:

_____
_____
_____

Start your day by watching a competition involving today's sport.

Math & Research Challenge

An official ping pong ball has a diameter of 40mm.

What is the surface area of an official ping pong ball?

Solve the challenge:

_____

_____

_____

_____

_____

_____

ANSWER:

_____

_____

Illustrate your answer:

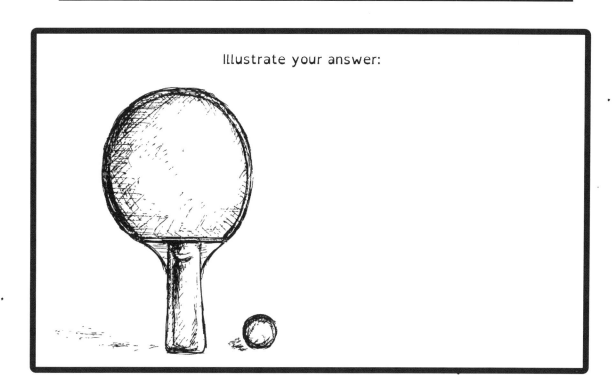

Sports Study

Ping Pong

It's research time!

Use the Internet, books, tutorials and documentaries to study this sport. Or go see a game or competition!

Draw any equipment needed for this sport.

Draw a player in uniform.

Draw a trophy or medal for this sport.

Where did this sport originate from?

_____

_____

How was this sport invented?

_____

_____

_____

Who are the main sponsors of the events for this sport?

_____

_____

What is the name of the largest competition where this sport is played? _____

_____

_____

_____

_____

Who is the #1 player of this sport? What makes them the best? How much money do they earn? Where do their earnings come from?

_____

_____

_____

_____

Would you like to play this sport? Why or why not?

_____

_____

What are the common injuries from playing this sport?

_____

_____

_____

Random fact about this sport.

_____

_____

_____

Say What?

Invent your own comic book font and add words to the picture

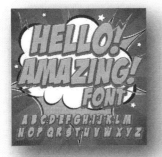
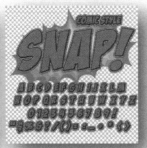
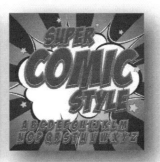
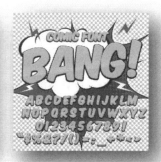

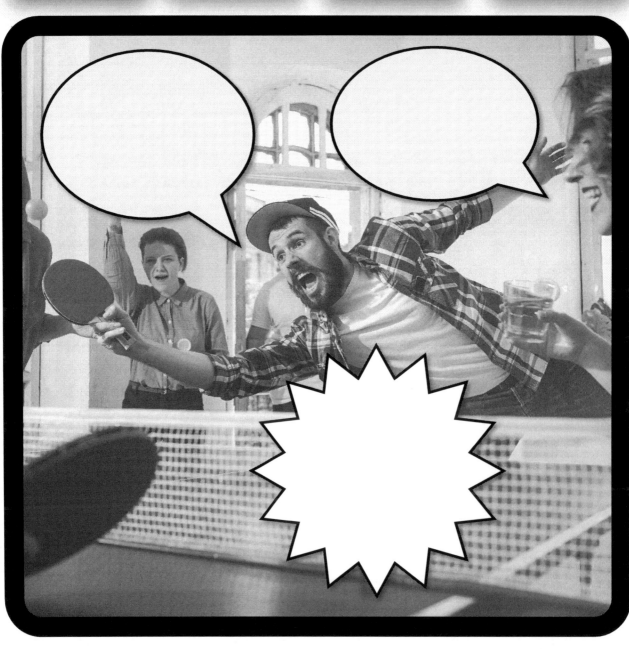

Sports News

Open a newspaper or look online!

What is happening in the world of sports today?

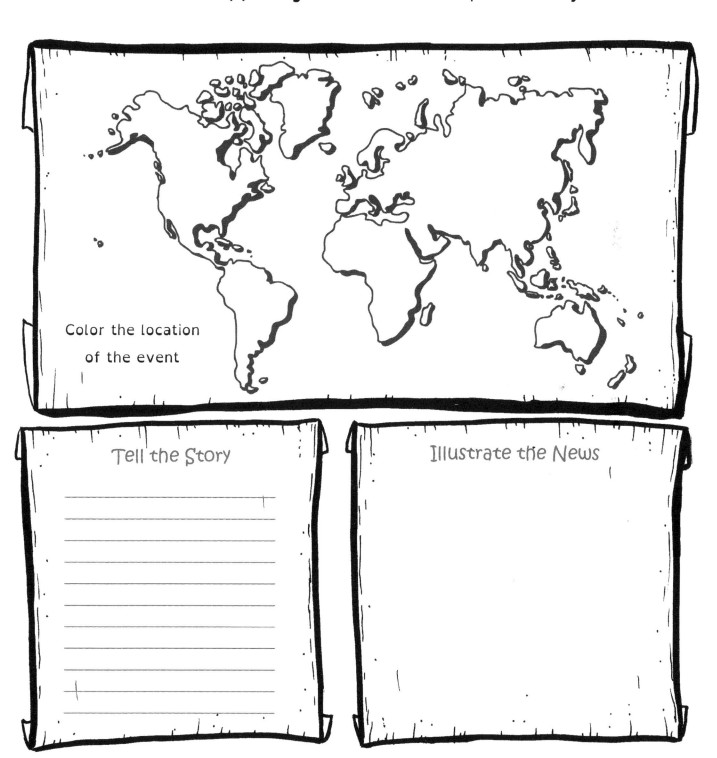

Color the location
of the event

Tell the Story

Illustrate the News

Screen Time

Watch a high-quality film, video, tutorial or sports documentary.

Title_____

Screen Time_____

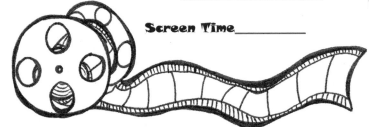

Producer_____

Actors_____

_____

_____

_____

Quotes

Draw a scene from the video.

Rating:

worst

Bad

Awful

Ok

Nice

Great

Best

Make a Comic

From the video or your imagination.

Title_____

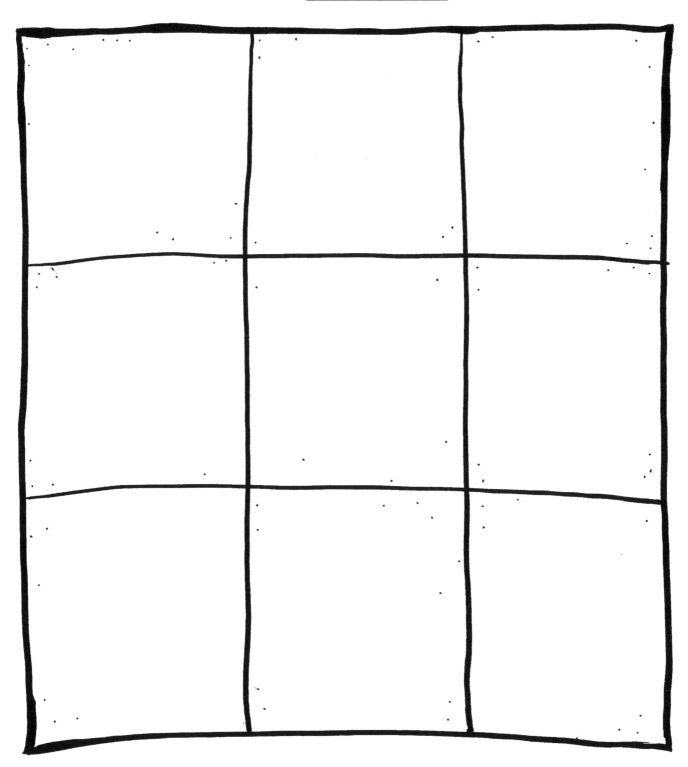

Drawing & Reading Time!

Choose a few books from your stack to focus on today.

Write down and draw anything that inspires you.

(Set a timer for 1 hour)

Free time!

Set the timer for 30 minutes and go outside to play, explore and practice a sport.

What do you plan to do on your free time?

_____

_____

What do you want to practice?

_____

_____

Do you have any goals?

_____

_____

Draw your goals!

Math Practice

Use this page for math practice,

or design a sport's field, rink or play zone

for the sport you are studying today!

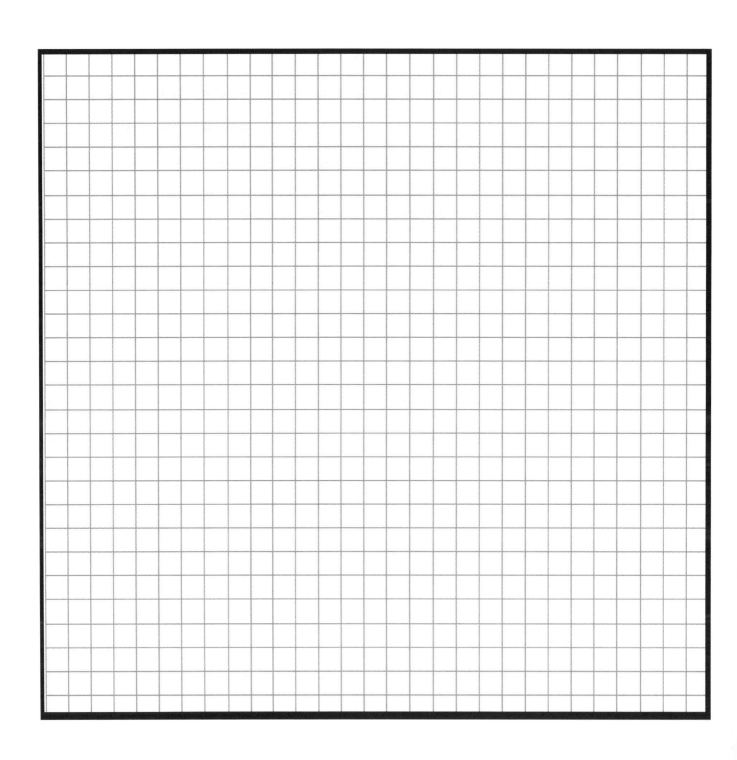

Nature Study

Take this book outside and draw anything and everything that inspires you.

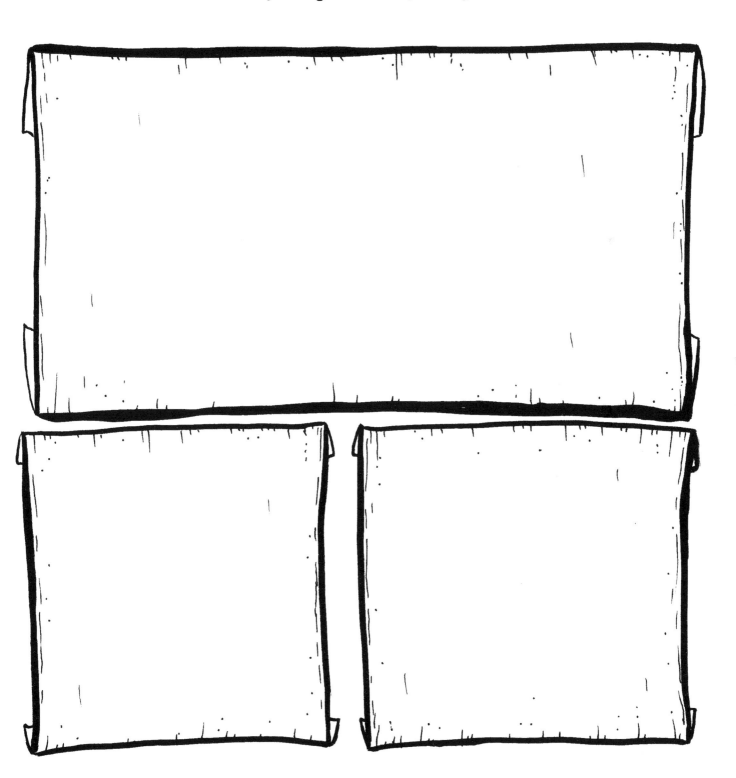

Today's Sport: Surfing

Date:_____

To-do List:

_____

_____

_____

_____

A Quote:

_____

_____

_____

_____

Today's Moods:

Today's Chores:

_____

_____

_____

_____

Books, Websites & Videos

Resources I can use to study today's sport:

_____

_____

_____

Start your day by watching a competition involving today's sport.

Math & Research Challenge

Surfers have a set amount of time in a competition to catch the best waves possible. The judges then take the top two wave scores and average them together for the surfer's final score. Mary has scores of 7.2, 8.5, 9.7, 3.4, 6.6, and 7.9. What was her final score?

Solve the challenge:

_____

_____

_____

_____

_____

_____

ANSWER:

_____

Illustrate your answer:

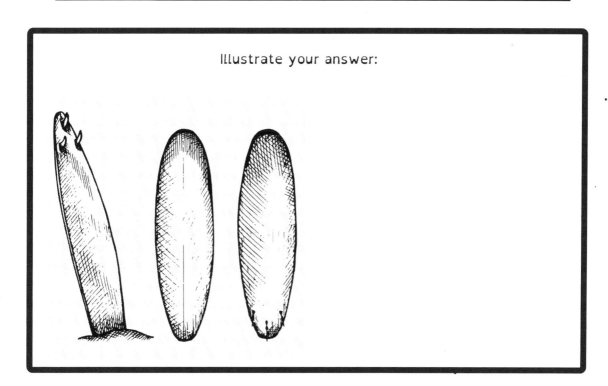

Surfing

It's research time!

Use the Internet, books, tutorials and documentaries to study this sport. Or go see a game or competition!

Draw any equipment needed for this sport.

Draw a player in uniform.

Draw a trophy or medal for this sport.

Where did this sport originate from?

_____

_____

How was this sport invented?

_____

_____

_____

Who are the main sponsors of the events for this sport?

_____

_____

What is the name of the largest competition where this sport is played? _____

_____

_____

_____

_____

Who is the #1 player of this sport? What makes them the best? How much money do they earn? Where do their earnings come from?

_____

_____

_____

_____

Would you like to play this sport? Why or why not?

_____

_____

_____

What are the common injuries from playing this sport?

_____

_____

_____

Random fact about this sport.

_____

_____

_____

Say What?

Invent your own comic book font and add words to the picture

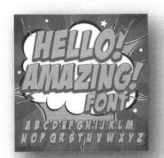
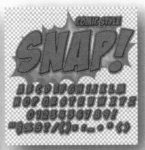
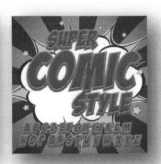
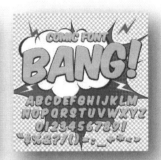

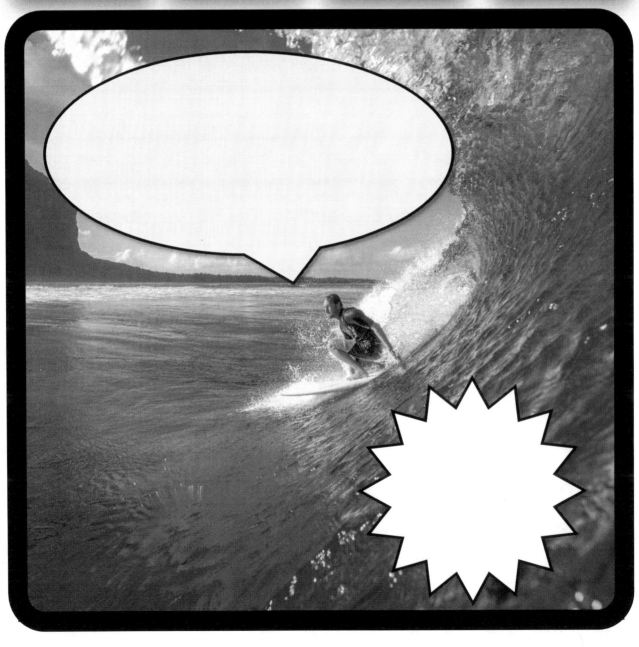

Sports News

Open a newspaper or look online!

What is happening in the world of sports today?

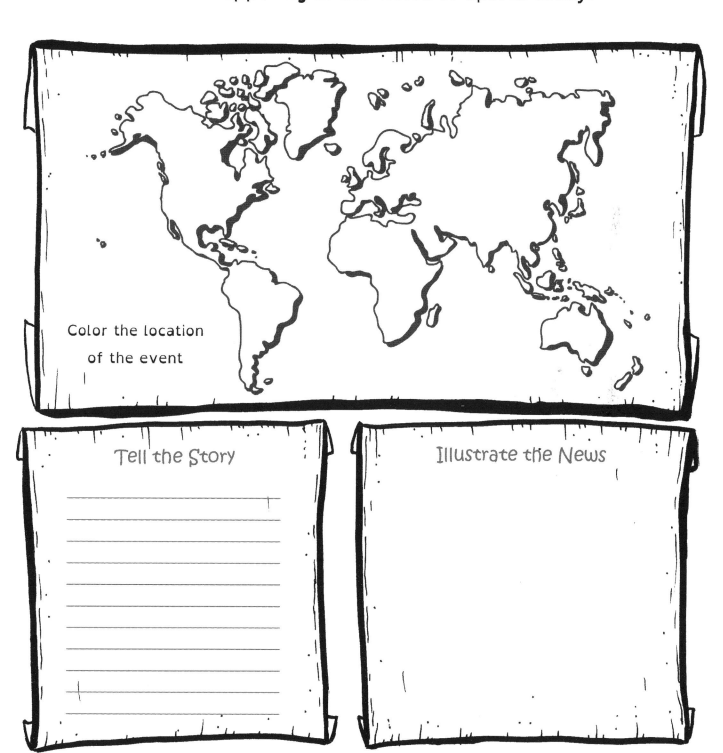

Color the location
of the event

Tell the Story

Illustrate the News

Screen Time

Watch a high-quality film, video, tutorial or sports documentary.

Title_____

Screen Time_____

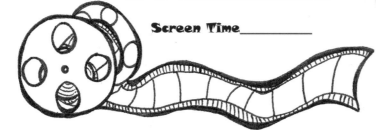

Producer_____

Actors_____

_____

_____

_____

Quotes

Draw a scene from the video.

Rating:

worst

Bad

Awful

Ok

Nice

Great

Best

Make a Comic

From the video or your imagination.

Title_____

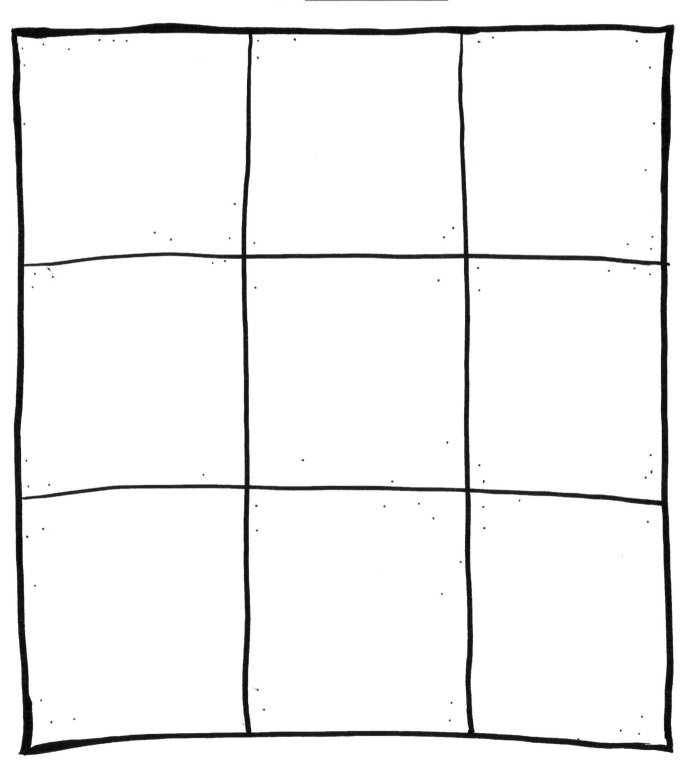

Drawing & Reading Time!

Choose a few books from your stack to focus on today.

Write down and draw anything that inspires you.

(Set a timer for 1 hour)

Free time!

Set the timer for 30 minutes and go outside to play,
explore and practice a sport.

What do you plan to do on your free time?

_____

_____

What do you want to practice?

_____

_____

Do you have any goals?

_____

_____

Draw your goals!

Math Practice

Use this page for math practice,

or design a sport's field, rink or play zone

for the sport you are studying today!

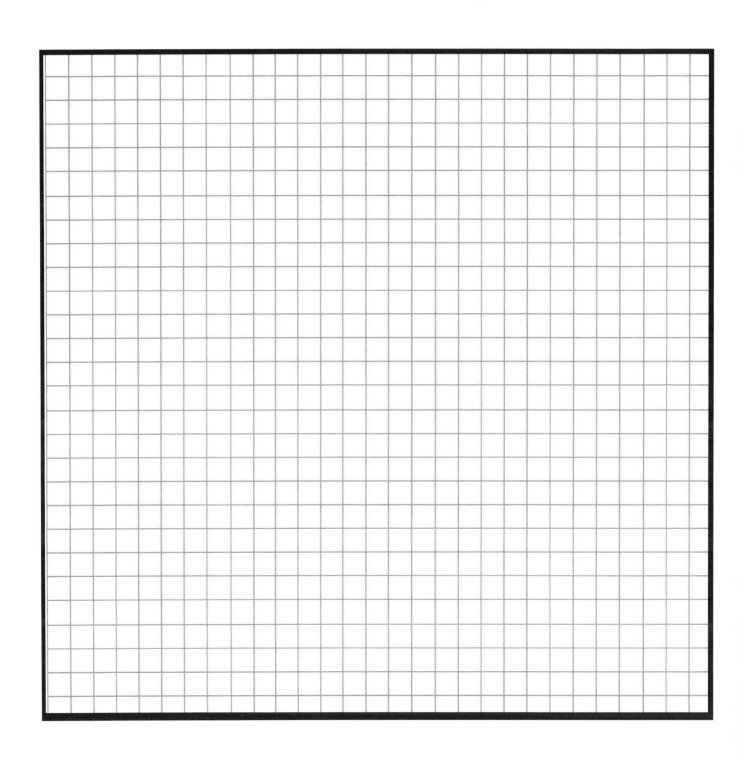

Nature Study

Take this book outside and draw anything and everything that inspires you.

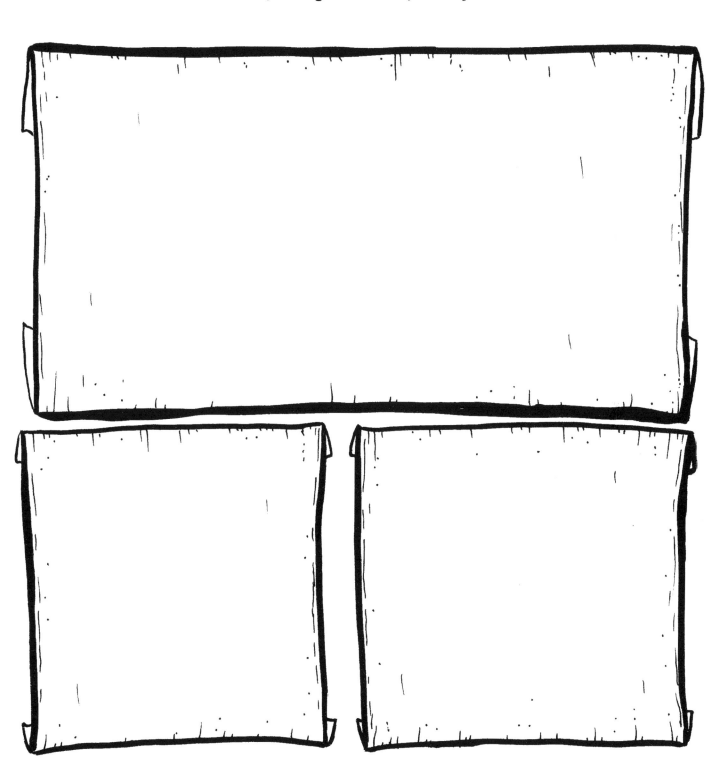

Today's Sport: Hiking

Date:_____

To-do List:

_____
_____
_____
_____

A Quote:

_____
_____
_____
_____

Today's Moods:

Today's Chores:

_____
_____
_____
_____

Books, Websites & Videos

Resources I can use to study today's sport:

_____
_____
_____

Start your day by watching a competition involving today's sport.

Math & Research Challenge

Sam and Kate are planning to hike the Appalachian Trail section of North Carolina and Tennessee in June. There are 95.7 miles of the Appalachian Trail in North Carolina, plus the Tennessee/North Carolina border for 224.7 additional miles. They will average 12 miles a day with a day off every 7 days. How many days will it take them to hike this section?

Solve the challenge:

_____
_____
_____
_____
_____
_____

ANSWER:

_____

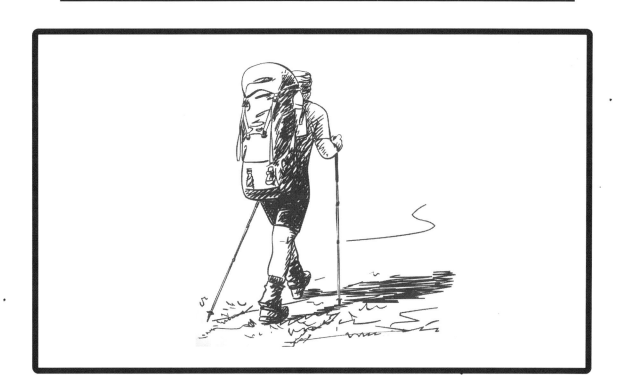

Hiking

It's research time!

Use the Internet, books, tutorials and documentaries to study this sport. Or go see a game or competition!

Draw any equipment needed for this sport.

Draw a player in uniform.

Draw a trophy or medal for this sport.

Where did this sport originate from?

_____

_____

How was this sport invented?

_____

_____

_____

Who are the main sponsors of the events for this sport?

_____

_____

What is the name of the largest competition where this sport is played? _____

_____

_____

_____

_____

Who is the #1 player of this sport? What makes them the best? How much money do they earn? Where do their earnings come from?

_____

_____

_____

_____

_____

Would you like to play this sport? Why or why not?

_____

_____

_____

What are the common injuries from playing this sport?

_____

_____

_____

_____

Random fact about this sport.

_____

_____

_____

Say What?

Invent your own comic book font and add words to the picture

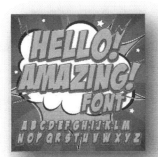
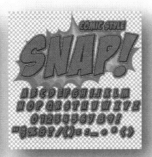
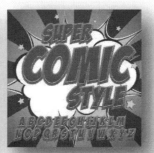
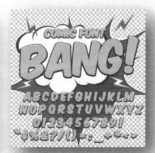

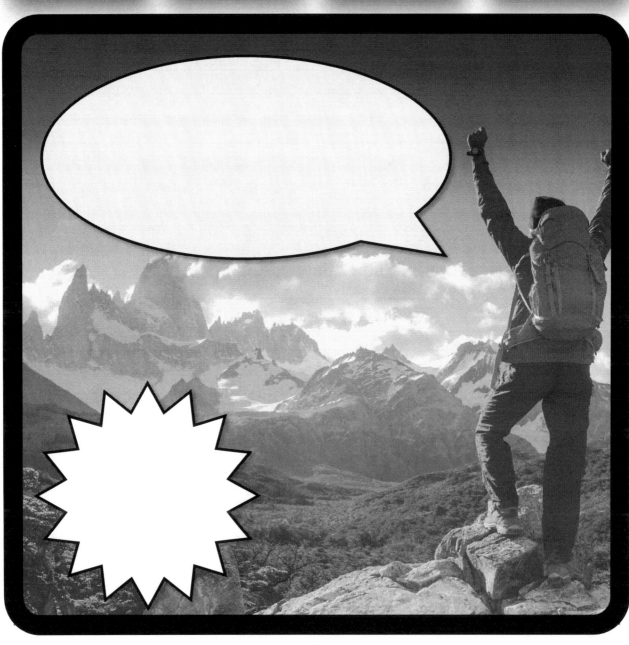

Sports News

Open a newspaper or look online!

What is happening in the world of sports today?

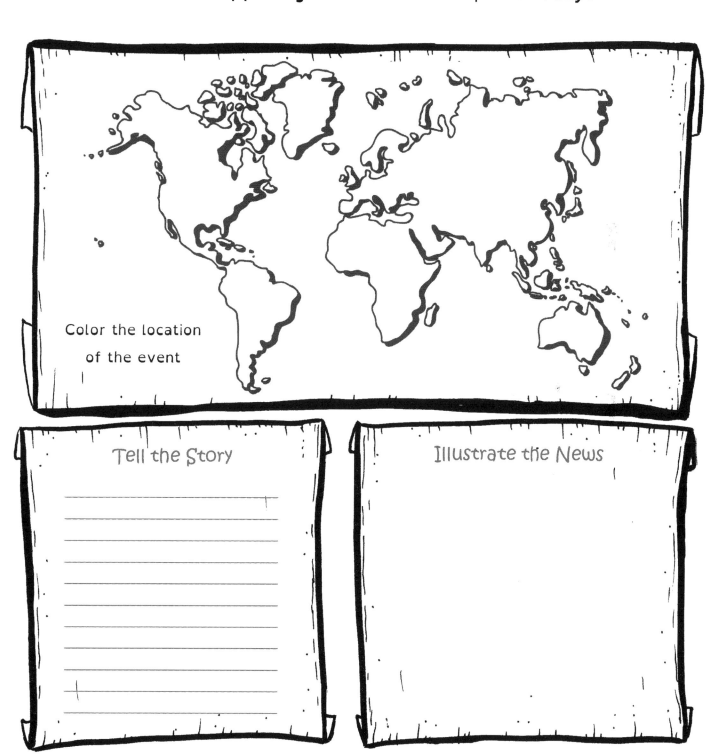

Color the location
of the event

Tell the Story

Illustrate the News

Screen Time

Watch a high-quality film, video, tutorial or sports documentary.

Title_____

Screen Time_____

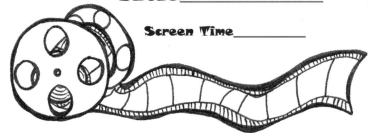

Producer_____

Actors_____

_____

_____

_____

Quotes

Draw a scene from the video.

Rating:

worst

Bad

Awful

Ok

Nice

Great

Best

Make a Comic

From the video or your imagination.

Title_____

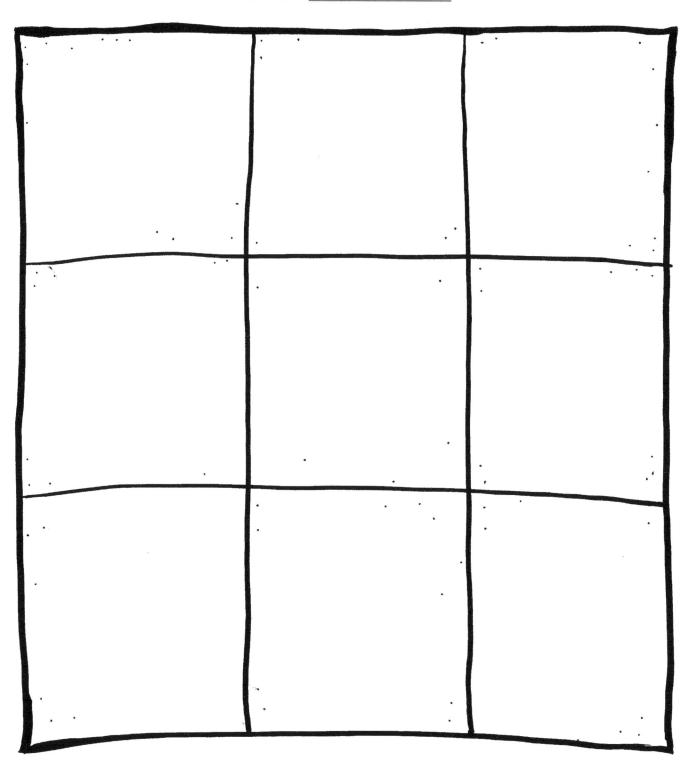

Drawing & Reading Time!

Choose a few books from your stack to focus on today.

Write down and draw anything that inspires you.

(Set a timer for 1 hour)

Free time!

Set the timer for 30 minutes and go outside to play, explore and practice a sport.

What do you plan to do on your free time?

_____

_____

What do you want to practice?

_____

_____

Do you have any goals?

_____

_____

Draw your goals!

Math Practice

Use this page for math practice,
or design a sport's field, rink or play zone
for the sport you are studying today!

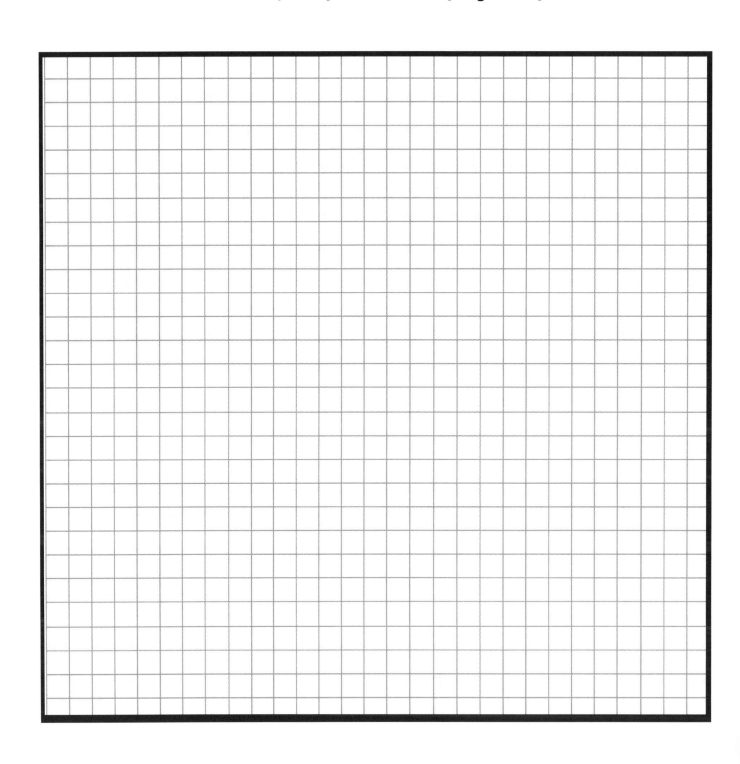

Nature Study

Take this book outside and draw anything and
everything that inspires you.

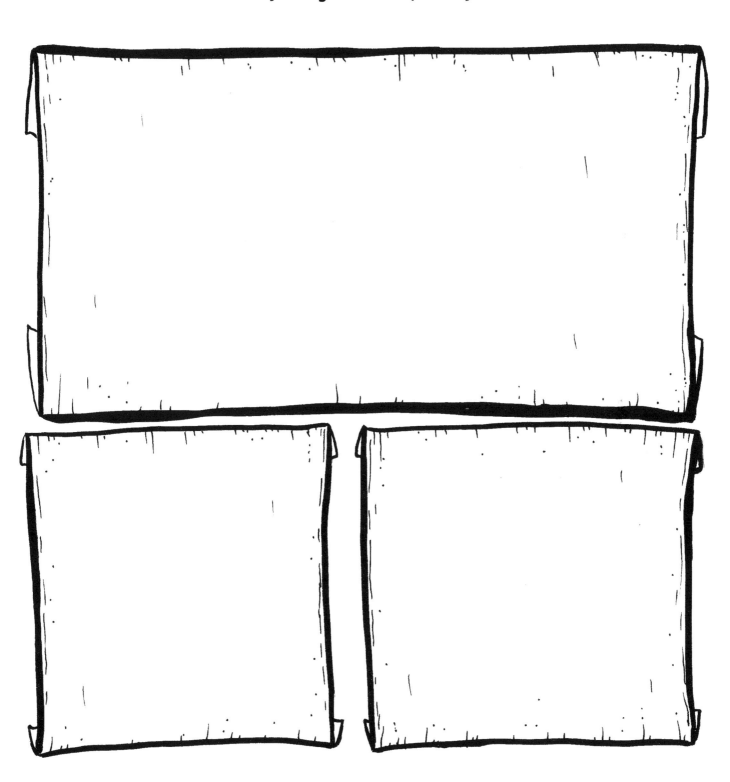

Today's Sport: Cricket

Date:_____

To-do List:

_____

_____

_____

_____

A Quote:

_____

_____

_____

_____

Today's Moods:

Today's Chores:

_____

_____

_____

_____

Books, Websites & Videos

Resources I can use to study today's sport:

_____

_____

_____

Start your day by watching a competition involving today's sport.

Math & Research Challenge

The records for most runs in an innings and most runs in a career are both held by Brian Lara of the West Indies. What was the score of his best game? Can you research and find the score of his most recent game and explain the difference between the two scores?

Solve the challenge:

_____

_____

_____

_____

_____

_____

ANSWER:

_____

Illustrate your answer:

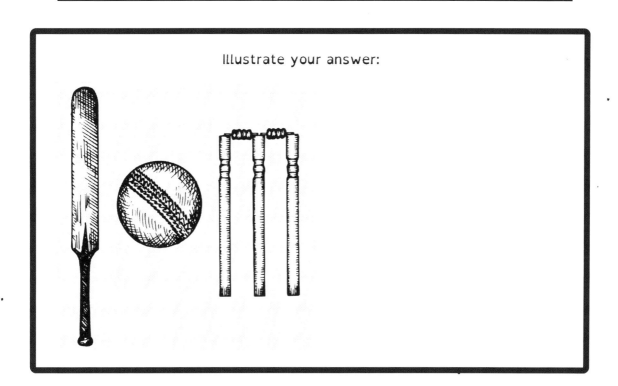

Sports Study

Cricket

It's research time!

Use the Internet, books, tutorials and documentaries to study
this sport. Or go see a game or competition!

Draw any equipment needed for this sport.

Draw a player in uniform.

Draw a trophy or medal for this sport.

Where did this sport originate from?

_____

_____

How was this sport invented?

_____

_____

_____

Who are the main sponsors of the events for this sport?

_____

_____

What is the name of the largest competition where this sport is played? _____

_____

_____

_____

_____

Who is the #1 player of this sport? What makes them the best? How much money do they earn? Where do their earnings come from?

_____

_____

_____

_____

Would you like to play this sport? Why or why not?

_____

_____

What are the common injuries from playing this sport?

_____

_____

_____

Random fact about this sport.

_____

_____

_____

Say What?

Invent your own comic book font and add words to the picture

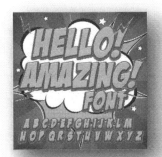
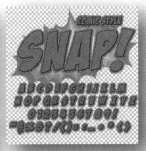
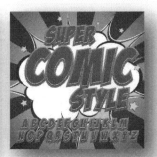
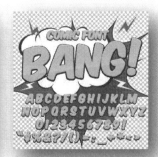

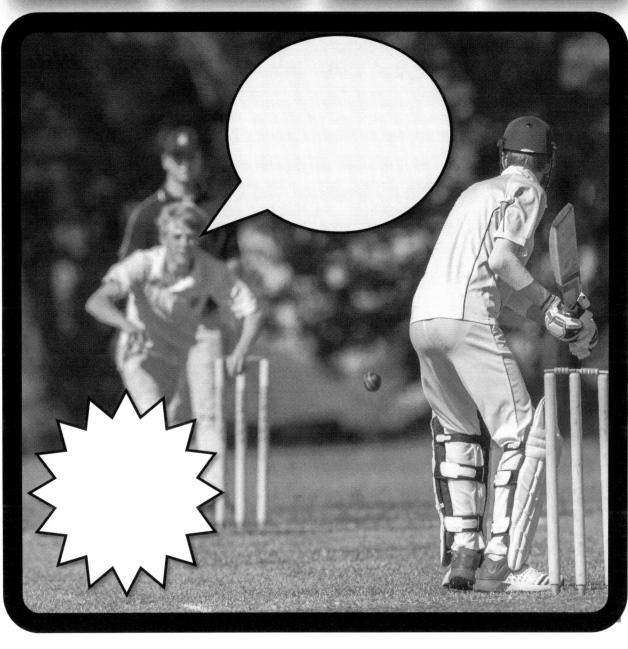

Sports News

Open a newspaper or look online!

What is happening in the world of sports today?

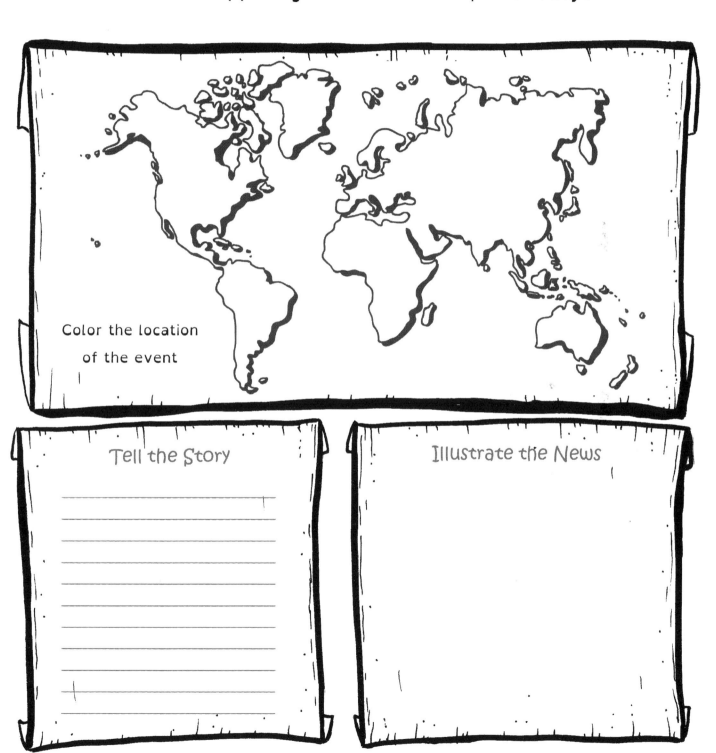

Color the location
of the event

Tell the Story

Illustrate the News

Screen Time

Watch a high-quality film, video, tutorial or sports documentary.

Title_____

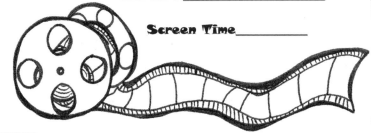

Screen Time_____

Producer_____

Actors_____

_____

_____

_____

Quotes

Draw a scene from the video.

Rating:

worst

Bad

Awful

Ok

Nice

Great

Best

Make a Comic

From the video or your imagination.

Title_____

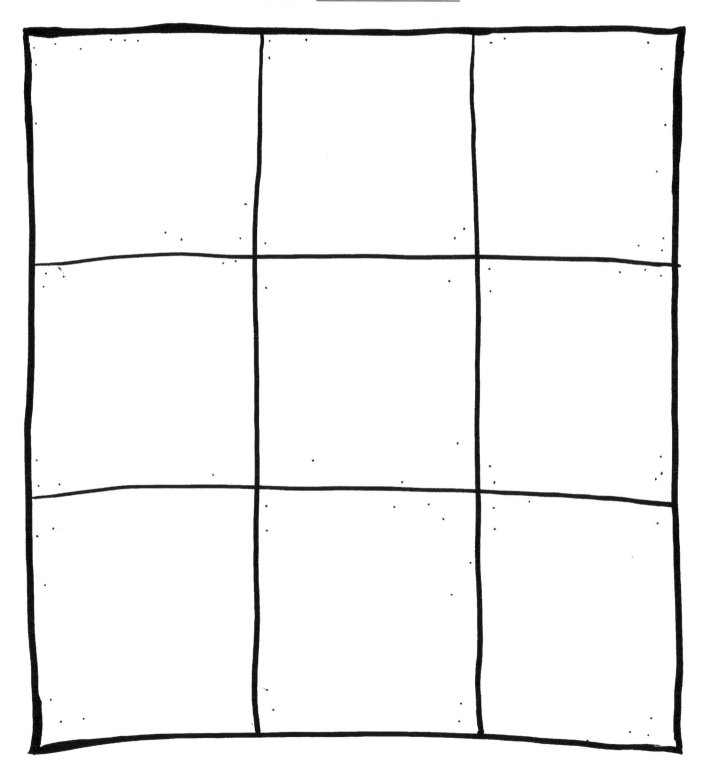

Drawing & Reading Time!

Choose a few books from your stack to focus on today.

Write down and draw anything that inspires you.

(Set a timer for 1 hour)

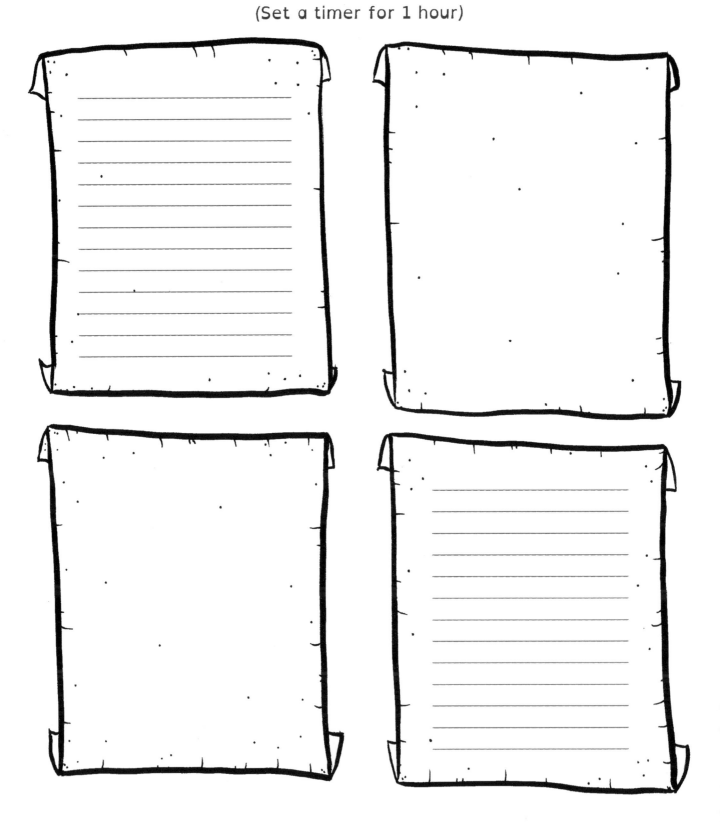

Free time!

Set the timer for 30 minutes and go outside to play, explore and practice a sport.

What do you plan to do on your free time?

_____

_____

What do you want to practice?

_____

_____

Do you have any goals?

_____

_____

Draw your goals!

Math Practice

Use this page for math practice,

or design a sport's field, rink or play zone

for the sport you are studying today!

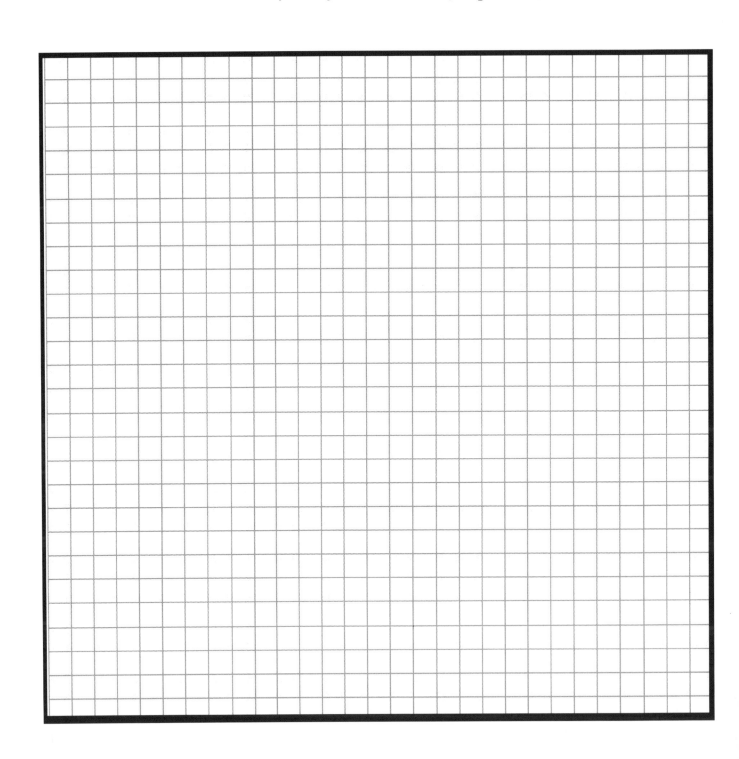

Nature Study

Take this book outside and draw anything and
everything that inspires you.

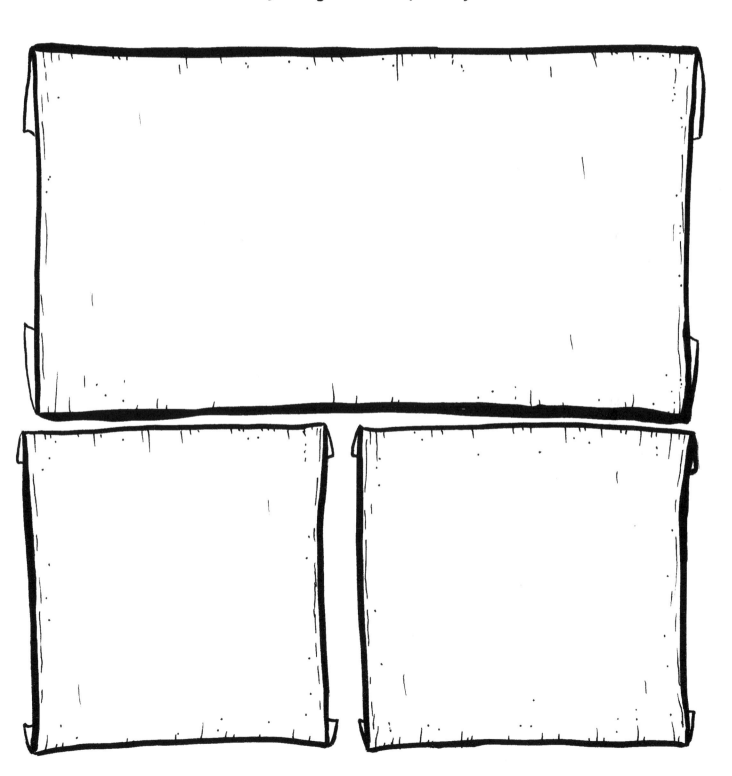

Today's Sport: Breakdancing

Date:_____

To-do List:

_____
_____
_____
_____

A Quote:

_____
_____
_____
_____

Today's Moods:

Today's Chores:

_____
_____
_____
_____

Books, Websites & Videos

Resources I can use to study today's sport:

_____
_____
_____

Start your day by watching a competition involving today's sport.

Finish the Story

Amber had been waiting years for this moment, since breakdancing was one of her strongest passion. After finding a team and practicing for hours on end, they were finally ready for the show. The lights dimmed and the music started...

_____

_____

_____

_____

_____

_____

_____

Illustrate your story:

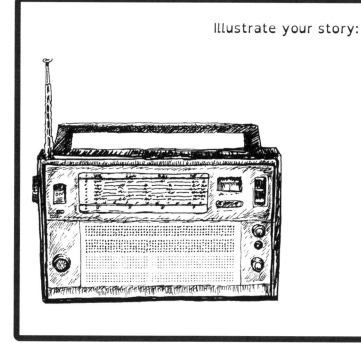

Breakdancing

It's research time!

Use the Internet, books, tutorials and documentaries to study this sport. Or go see a game or competition!

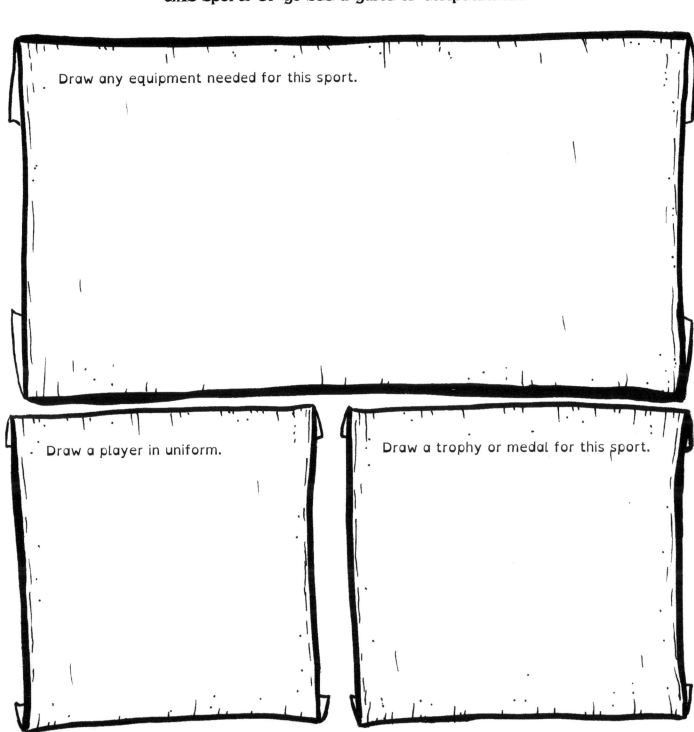

Draw any equipment needed for this sport.

Draw a player in uniform.

Draw a trophy or medal for this sport.

Where did this sport originate from?

_____

_____

How was this sport invented?

_____

_____

_____

Who are the main sponsors of the events for this sport?

_____

_____

What is the name of the largest competition where this sport is played? _____

_____

_____

_____

_____

Who is the #1 player of this sport? What makes them the best? How much money do they earn? Where do their earnings come from?

_____

_____

_____

_____

Would you like to play this sport? Why or why not?

_____

_____

_____

What are the common injuries from playing this sport?

_____

_____

_____

_____

Random fact about this sport.

_____

_____

_____

Say What?

Invent your own comic book font and add words to the picture

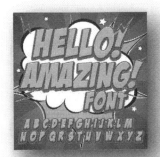
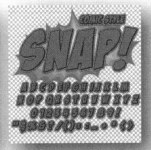
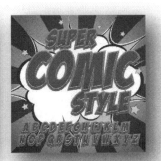
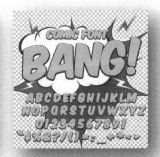

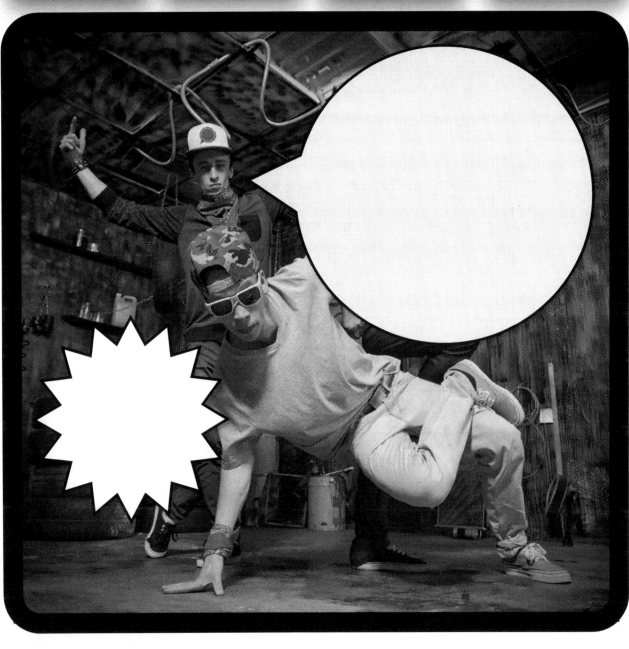

Sports News

Open a newspaper or look online!

What is happening in the world of sports today?

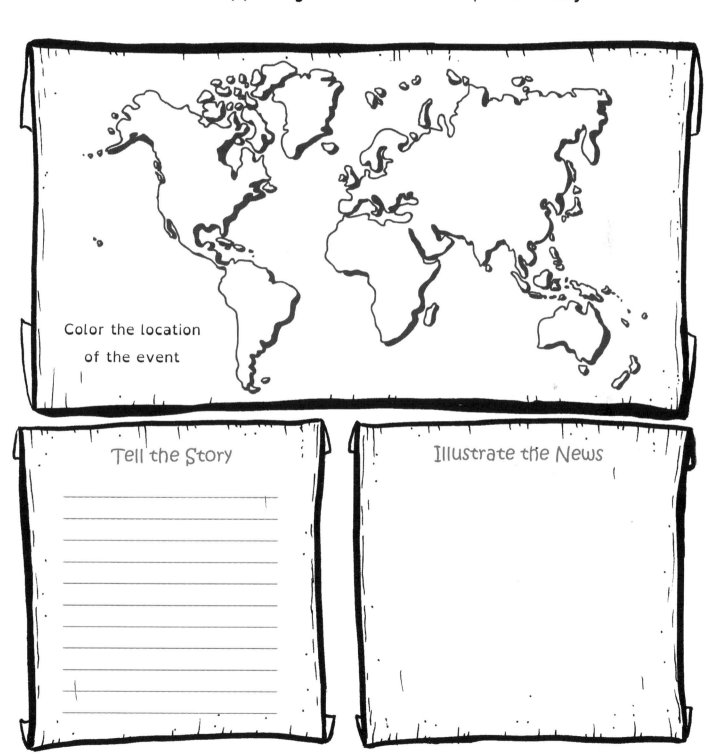

Color the location
of the event

Tell the Story

Illustrate the News

Screen Time

Watch a high-quality film, video, tutorial or sports documentary.

Title_____

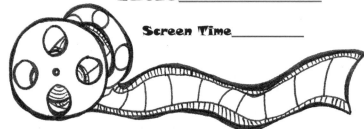

Screen Time_____

Producer_____

Actors_____

_____

_____

_____

Quotes

Draw a scene from the video.

Rating:

worst

Bad

Awful

Ok

Nice

Great

Best

Make a Comic

From the video or your imagination.

Title_____

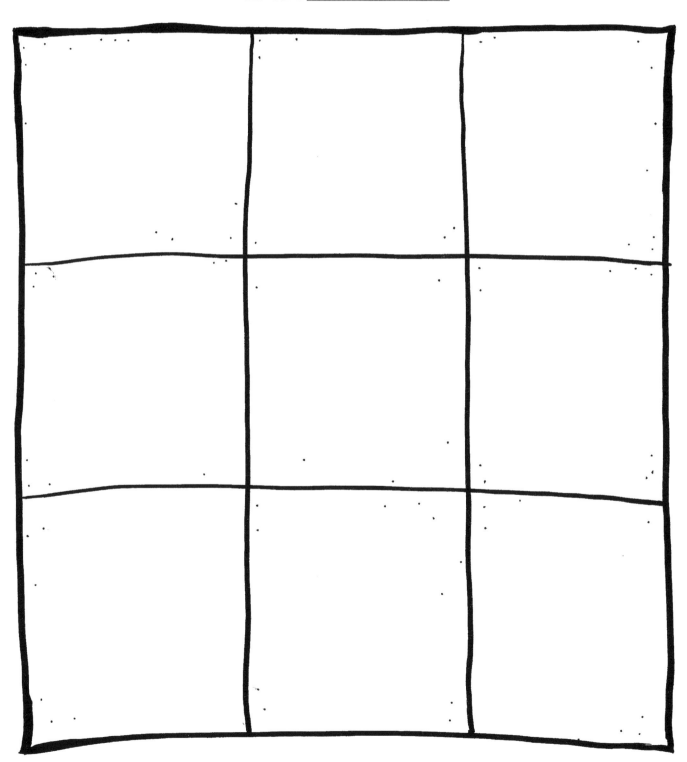

Drawing & Reading Time!

Choose a few books from your stack to focus on today.

Write down and draw anything that inspires you.

(Set a timer for 1 hour)

Free time!

Set the timer for 30 minutes and go outside to play,
explore and practice a sport.

What do you plan to do on your free time?

_____

_____

What do you want to practice?

_____

_____

Do you have any goals?

_____

_____

Draw your goals!

Math Practice

Use this page for math practice,

or design a sport's field, rink or play zone

for the sport you are studying today!

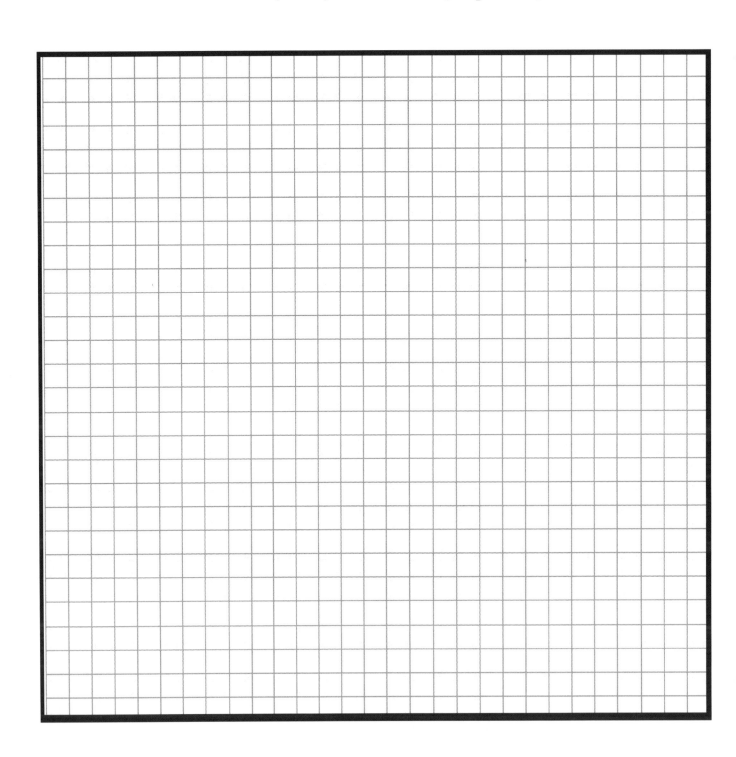

Nature Study

Take this book outside and draw anything and everything that inspires you.

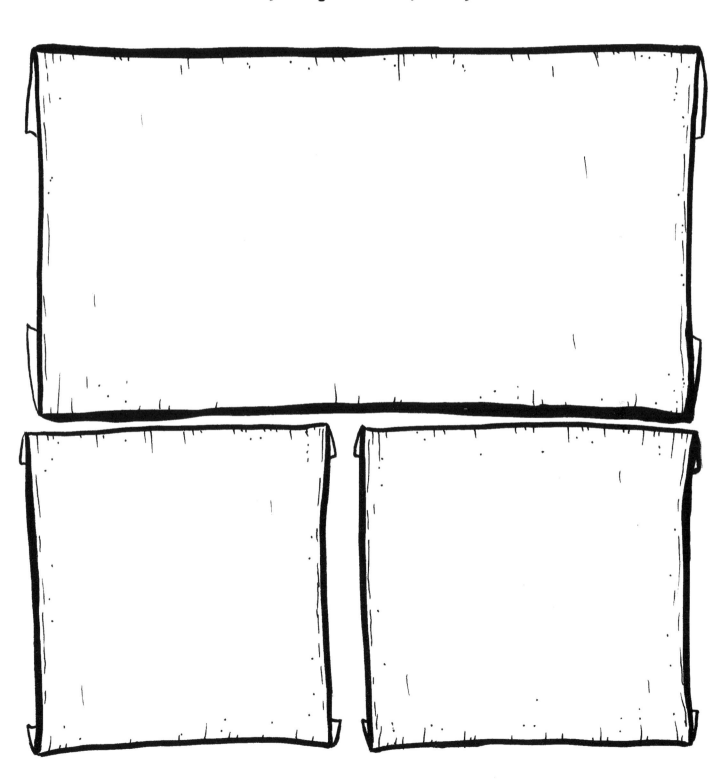

Today's Sport: Cycling

Date:_____

To-do List:
_____
_____
_____
_____

A Quote:
_____
_____
_____
_____
_____

Today's Moods:

Today's Chores:
_____
_____
_____
_____

Books, Websites & Videos

Resources I can use to study today's sport:

_____
_____
_____

Start your day by watching a competition involving today's sport.

Math & Research Challenge

You are planning a cycling trip to the Alpine Pass Cycle Tour in France. The tour runs from St. Michel de Maurienne to Grasse and is 325 kilometers long. Convert the distance you will travel into miles.

Solve the challenge:

_____
_____
_____
_____
_____
_____

ANSWER:

_____

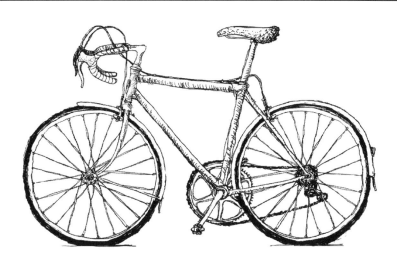

Bonus - Look up the route and plan a trip.
Where will you stop and what you will bring?

Sports Study

Cycling

It's research time!

Use the Internet, books, tutorials and documentaries to study
this sport. Or go see a game or competition!

Draw any equipment needed for this sport.

Draw a player in uniform.

Draw a trophy or medal for this sport.

Where did this sport originate from?

_____

_____

How was this sport invented?

_____

_____

_____

Who are the main sponsors of the events for this sport?

_____

_____

What is the name of the largest competition where this sport is played? _____

_____

_____

_____

Who is the #1 player of this sport? What makes them the best? How much money do they earn? Where do their earnings come from?

_____

_____

_____

_____

Would you like to play this sport? Why or why not?

_____

_____

_____

What are the common injuries from playing this sport?

_____

_____

_____

Random fact about this sport.

_____

_____

_____

Say What?

Invent your own comic book font and add words to the picture

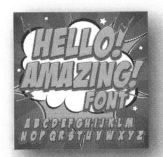
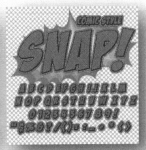
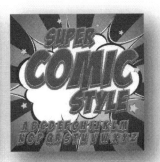
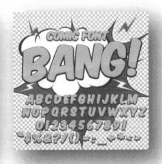

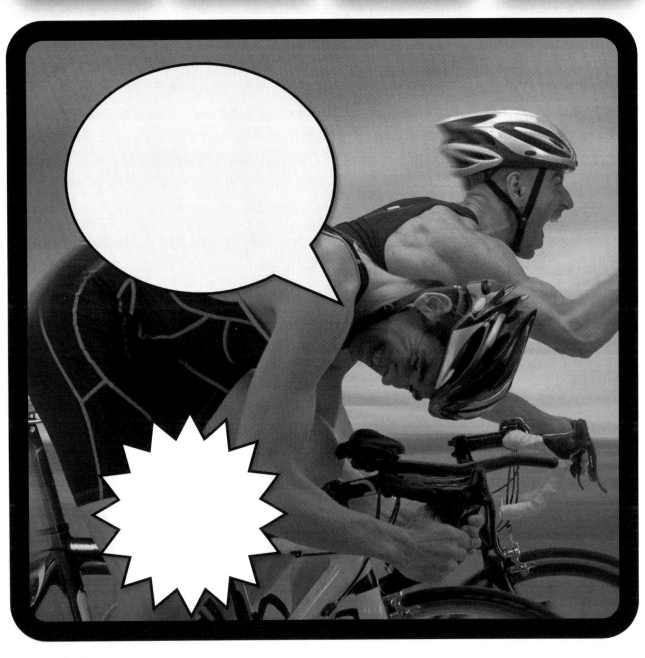

Sports News

Open a newspaper or look online!

What is happening in the world of sports today?

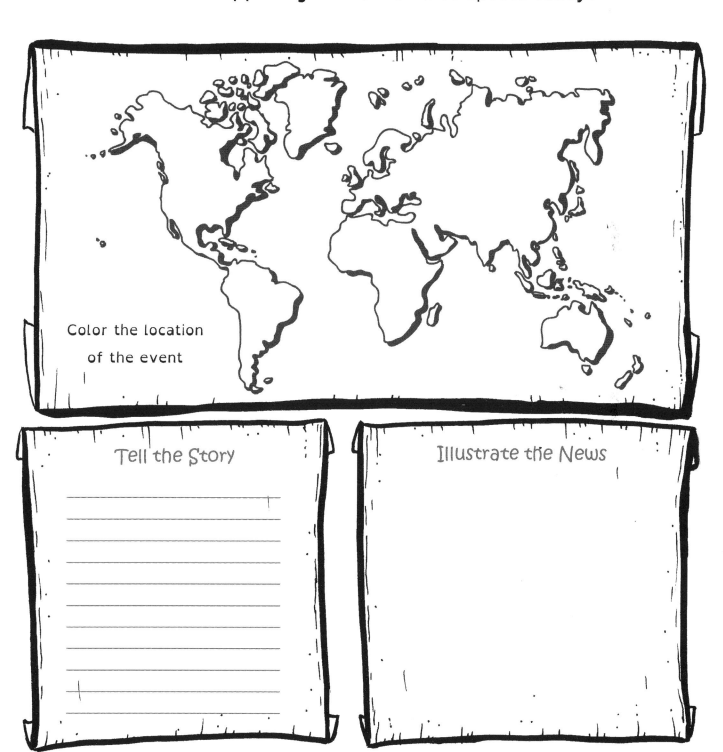

Color the location
of the event

Tell the Story

Illustrate the News

Screen Time

Watch a high-quality film, video, tutorial or sports documentary.

Title_____

Screen Time_____

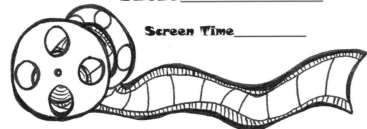

Producer_____

Actors_____

_____

_____

_____

Quotes

Draw a scene from the video.

Rating:

worst

Bad

Awful

Ok

Nice

Great

Best

Make a Comic

From the video or your imagination.

Title_____

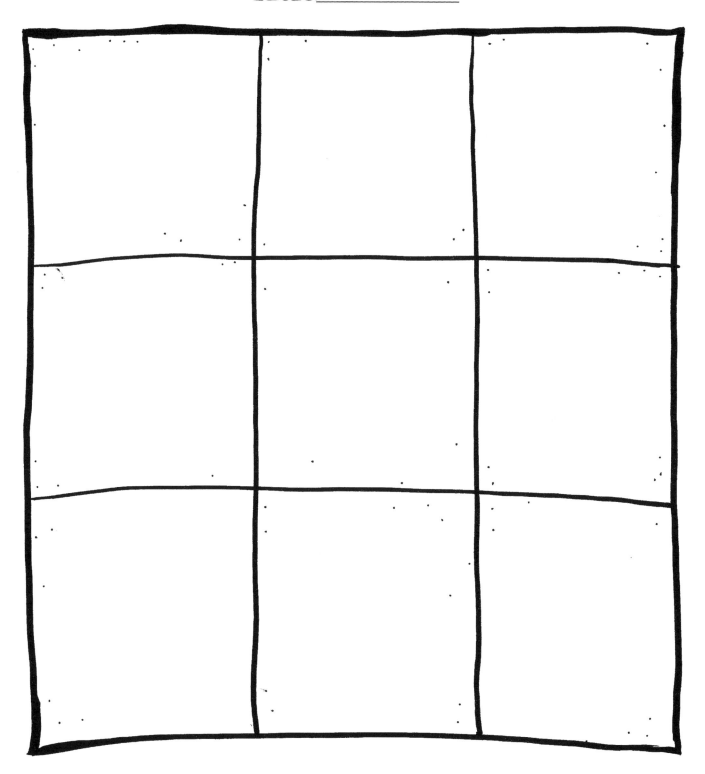

Drawing & Reading Time!

Choose a few books from your stack to focus on today.

Write down and draw anything that inspires you.

(Set a timer for 1 hour)

Free time!

Set the timer for 30 minutes and go outside to play,
explore and practice a sport.

What do you plan to do on your free time?

What do you want to practice?

Do you have any goals?

Draw your goals!

Math Practice

Use this page for math practice,

or design a sport's field, rink or play zone

for the sport you are studying today!

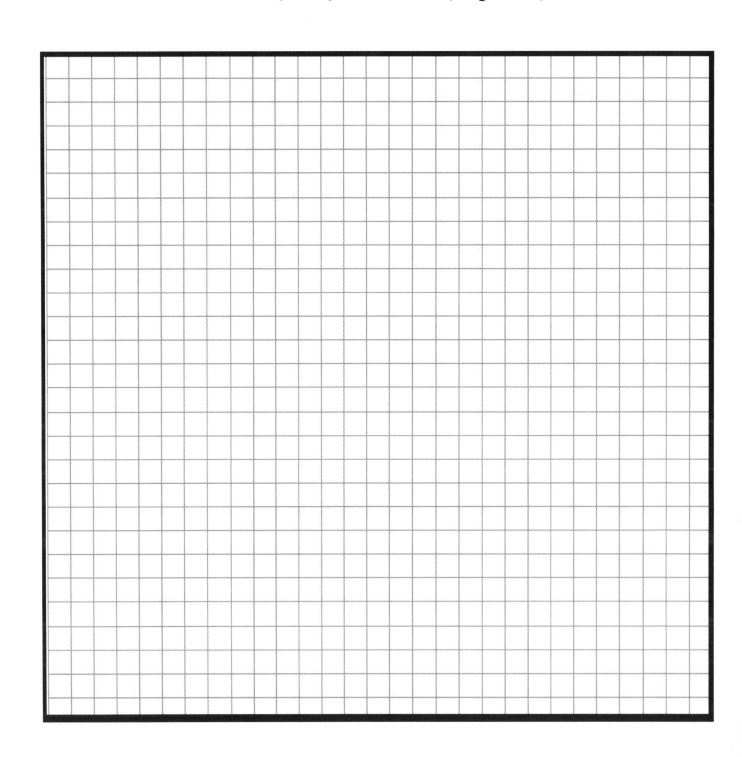

Nature Study

Take this book outside and draw anything and everything that inspires you.

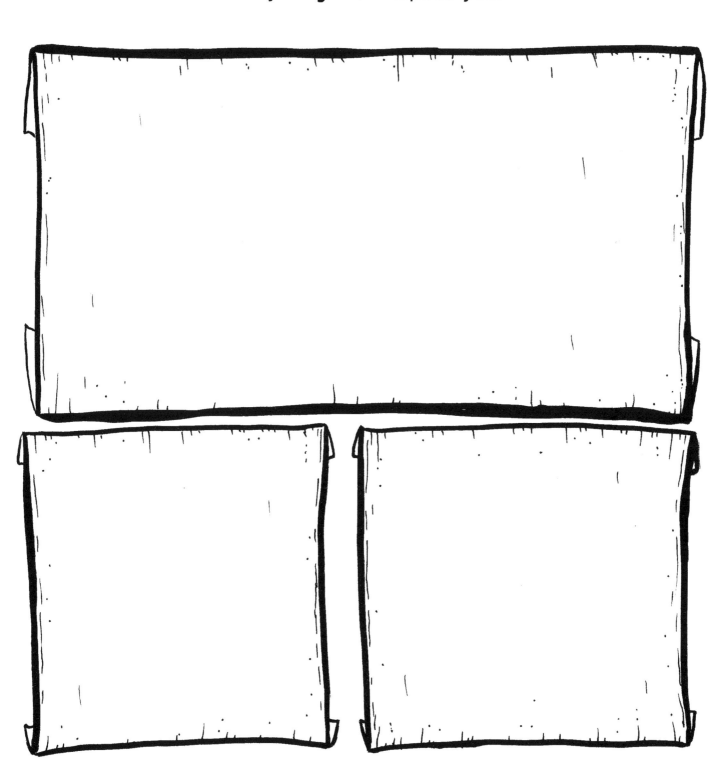

Today's Sport: Boxing

Date:_____

To-do List:

_____
_____
_____
_____

A Quote:

_____
_____
_____
_____

Today's Moods:

Today's Chores:

_____
_____
_____
_____

Books, Websites & Videos

Resources I can use to study today's sport:

_____
_____
_____

Start your day by watching a competition involving today's sport.

Math & Research Challenge

A professional boxing match takes place over 12 three minute rounds with a one minute break in between rounds. How many minutes pass from the beginning of the match until the end of the twelfth round?

Solve the challenge:

_____
_____
_____
_____
_____
_____

ANSWER:

_____

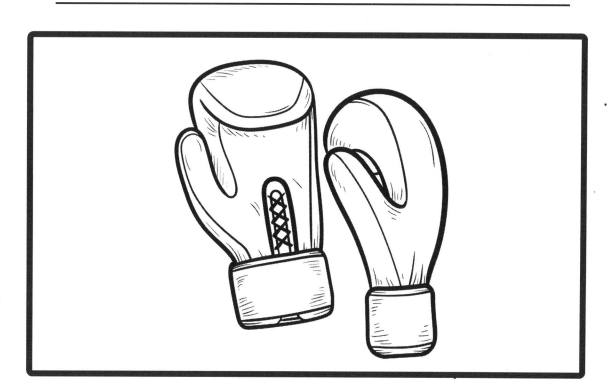

Boxing

It's research time!

Use the Internet, books, tutorials and documentaries to study this sport. Or go see a game or competition!

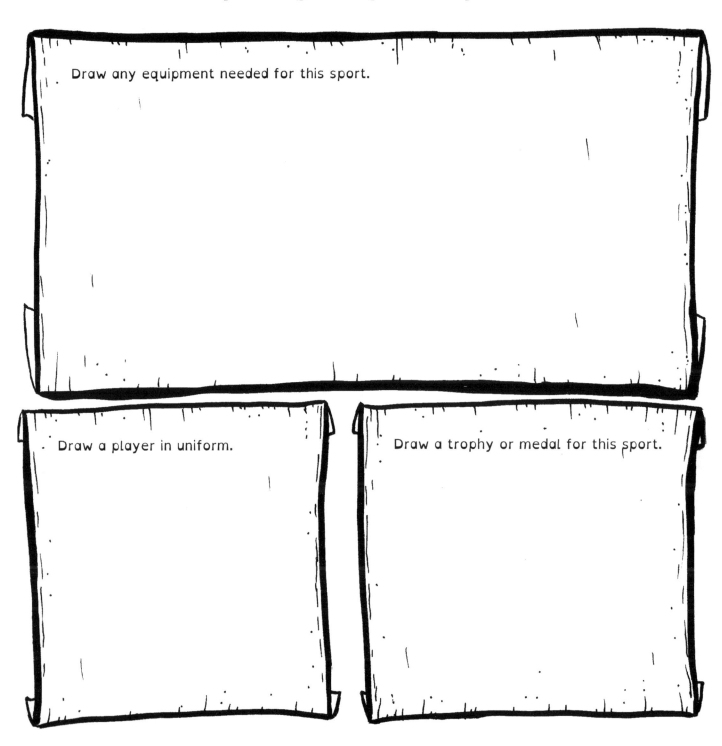

Draw any equipment needed for this sport.

Draw a player in uniform.

Draw a trophy or medal for this sport.

Where did this sport originate from?

_____

_____

How was this sport invented?

_____

_____

_____

Who are the main sponsors of the events for this sport?

_____

_____

What is the name of the largest competition where this sport is played? _____

_____

_____

_____

_____

Who is the #1 player of this sport? What makes them the best? How much money do they earn? Where do their earnings come from?

_____

_____

_____

_____

_____

Would you like to play this sport? Why or why not?

_____

_____

_____

What are the common injuries from playing this sport?

_____

_____

_____

_____

Random fact about this sport.

_____

_____

_____

Say What?

Invent your own comic book font and add words to the picture

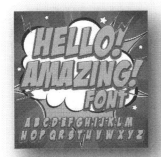
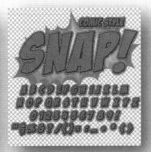
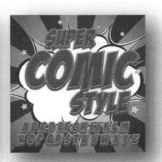
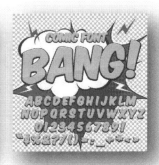

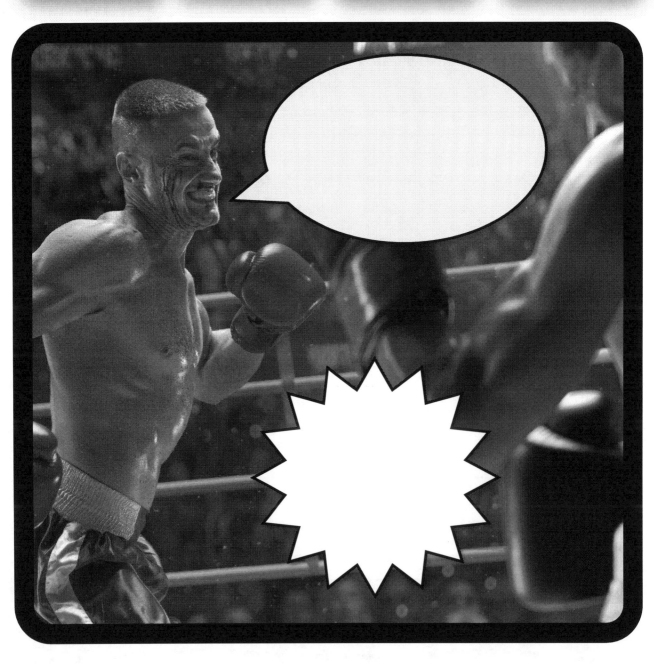

Sports News

Open a newspaper or look online!

What is happening in the world of sports today?

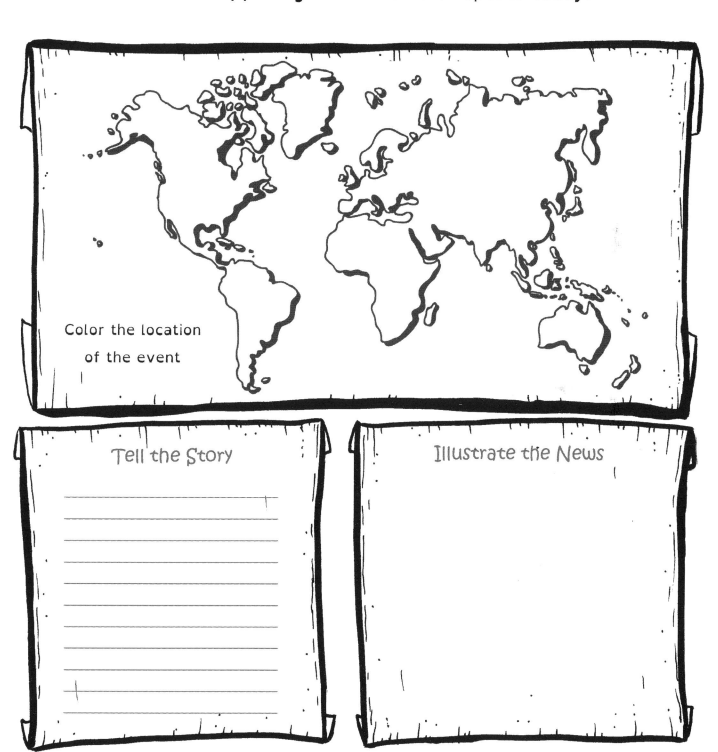

Color the location
of the event

Tell the Story

Illustrate the News

Screen Time

Watch a high-quality film, video, tutorial or sports documentary.

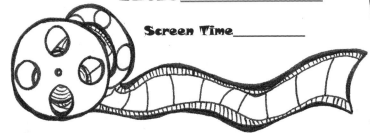

Title_____

Screen Time_____

Producer_____

Actors_____

_____

_____

_____

Quotes

Draw a scene from the video.

Rating:

worst

Bad

Awful

Ok

Nice

Great

Best

Make a Comic

From the video or your imagination.

Title_____

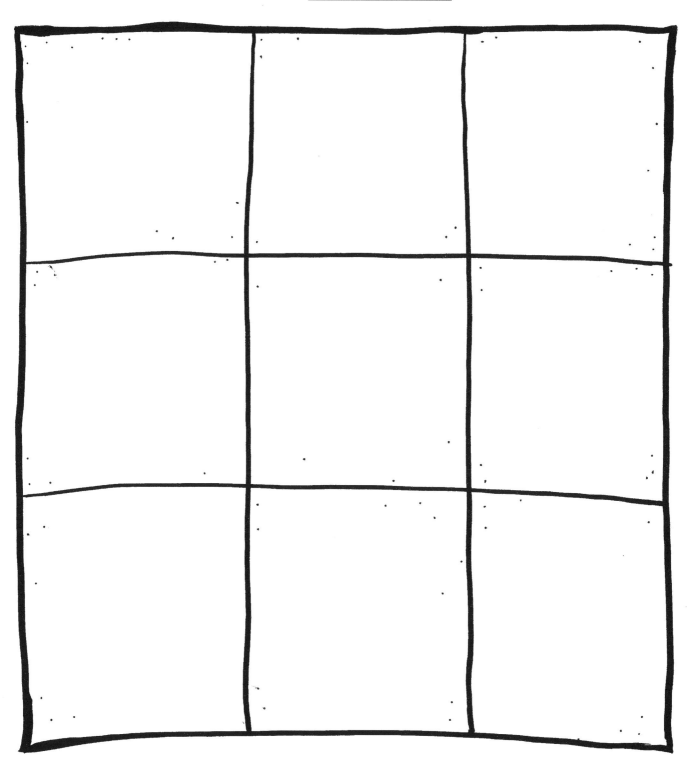

Drawing & Reading Time!

Choose a few books from your stack to focus on today.

Write down and draw anything that inspires you.

(Set a timer for 1 hour)

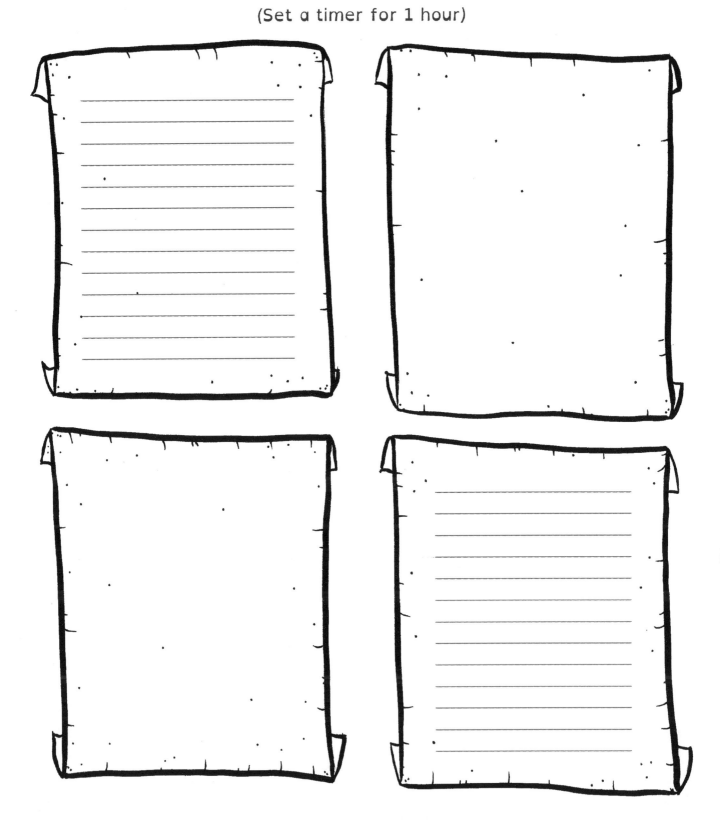

Free time!

Set the timer for 30 minutes and go outside to play, explore and practice a sport.

What do you plan to do on your free time?

What do you want to practice?

Do you have any goals?

Draw your goals!

Math Practice

Use this page for math practice,
or design a sport's field, rink or play zone
for the sport you are studying today!

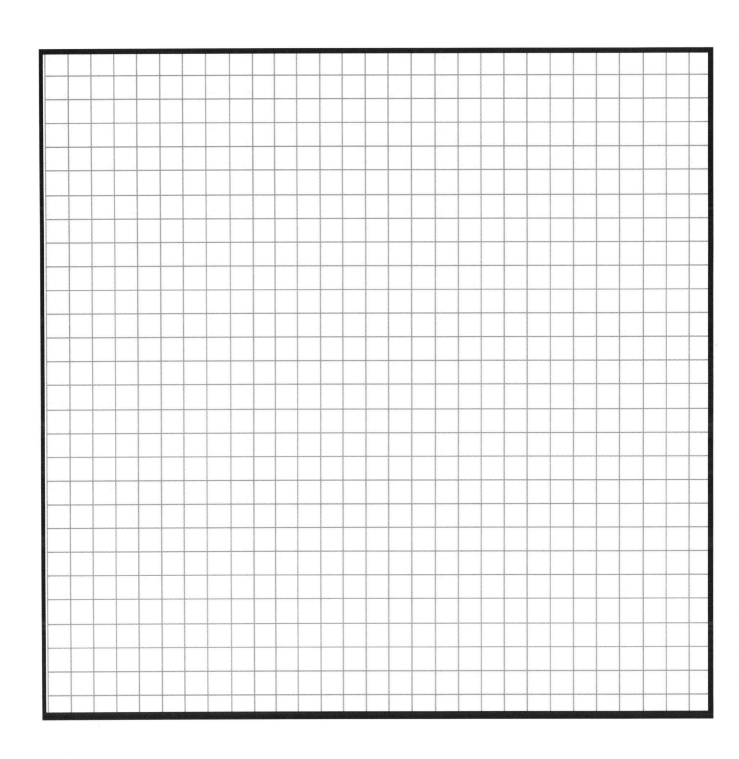

Nature Study

Take this book outside and draw anything and
everything that inspires you.

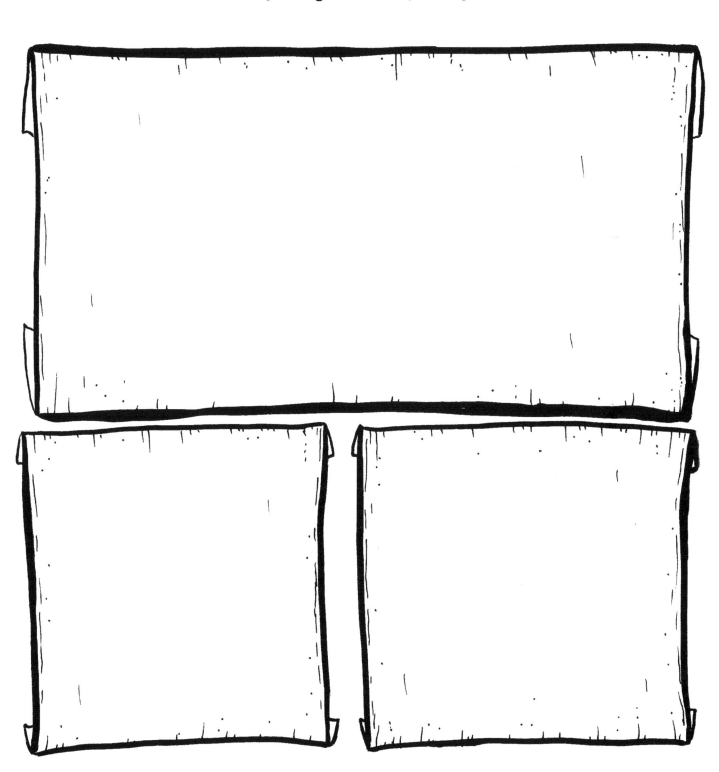

Today's Sport: Baseball

Date:_____

To-do List:

_____
_____
_____
_____

A Quote:

_____
_____
_____
_____

Today's Moods:

Today's Chores:

_____
_____
_____
_____

Books, Websites & Videos

Resources I can use to study today's sport:

_____
_____
_____

Start your day by watching a competition involving today's sport.

Finish the Story

The bases are loaded with Darren up to bat. It's the bottom of the ninth with two outs. The crowd is cheering! Trenton on third base nervously waits for the pitch. The pitcher throws the ball. Darren swings...

_____

_____

_____

_____

_____

_____

_____

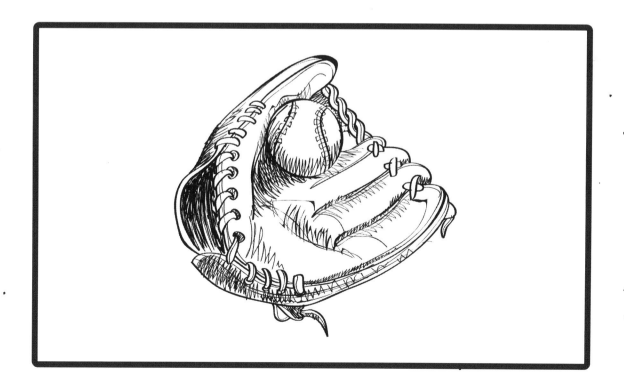

Sports Study

Baseball

It's research time!

Use the Internet, books, tutorials and documentaries to study
this sport. Or go see a game or competition!

Draw any equipment needed for this sport.

Draw a player in uniform.

Draw a trophy or medal for this sport.

Where did this sport originate from?

_____

_____

How was this sport invented?

_____

_____

_____

Who are the main sponsors of the events for this sport?

_____

_____

What is the name of the largest competition where this sport is played? _____

_____

_____

_____

_____

Who is the #1 player of this sport? What makes them the best? How much money do they earn? Where do their earnings come from?

_____

_____

_____

_____

Would you like to play this sport? Why or why not?

_____

_____

What are the common injuries from playing this sport?

_____

_____

_____

_____

Random fact about this sport.

_____

_____

_____

Say What?

Invent your own comic book font and add words to the picture

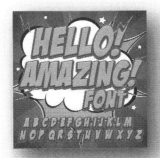
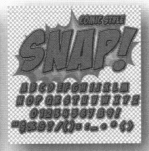
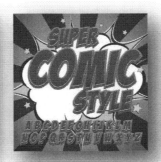
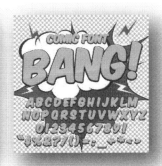

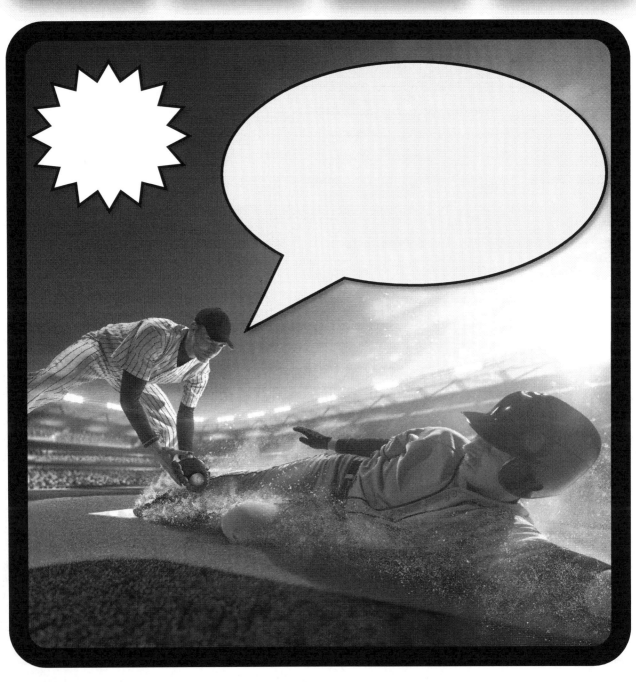

Sports News

Open a newspaper or look online!

What is happening in the world of sports today?

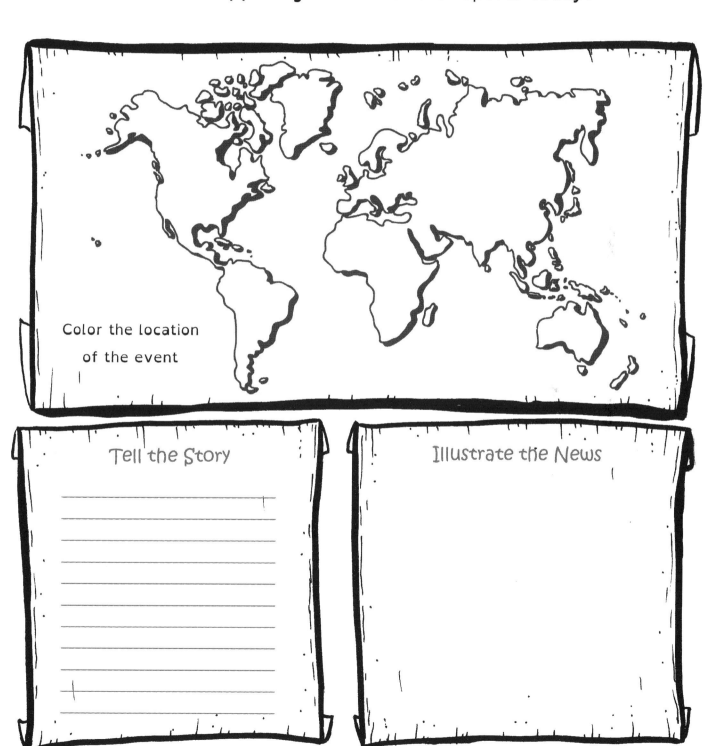

Color the location
of the event

Tell the Story

Illustrate the News

Screen Time

Watch a high-quality film, video, tutorial or sports documentary.

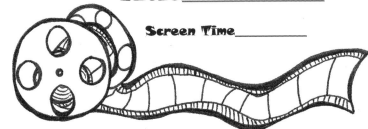

Title_____

Screen Time_____

Producer_____

Actors_____

_____

_____

_____

Quotes

Draw a scene from the video.

Rating:

worst

Bad

Awful

Ok

Nice

Great

Best

Make a Comic

From the video or your imagination.

Title_____

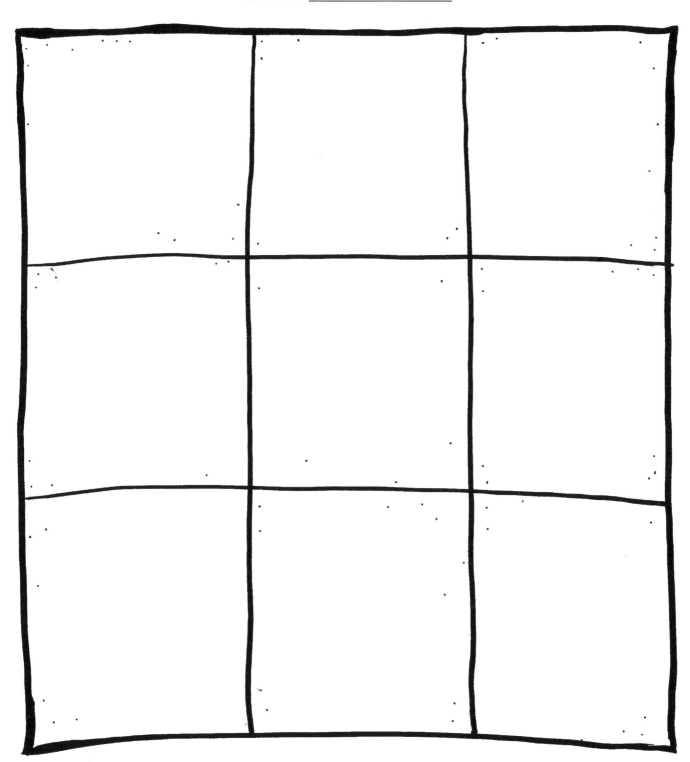

Drawing & Reading Time!

Choose a few books from your stack to focus on today.

Write down and draw anything that inspires you.

(Set a timer for 1 hour)

Free time!

Set the timer for 30 minutes and go outside to play, explore and practice a sport.

What do you plan to do on your free time?

_____

_____

What do you want to practice?

_____

_____

Do you have any goals?

_____

_____

Draw your goals!

Math Practice

Use this page for math practice,
or design a sport's field, rink or play zone
for the sport you are studying today!

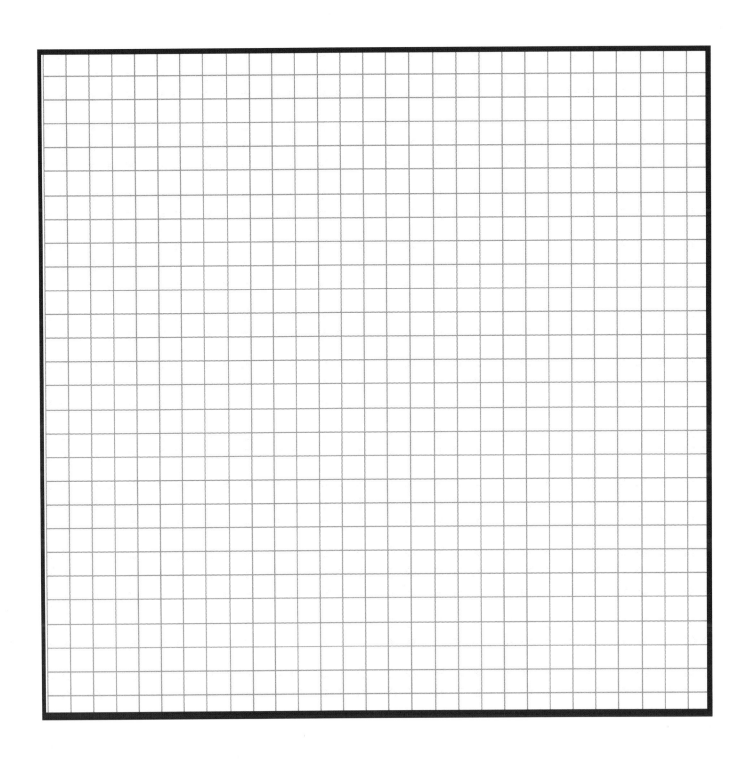

Nature Study

Take this book outside and draw anything and
everything that inspires you.

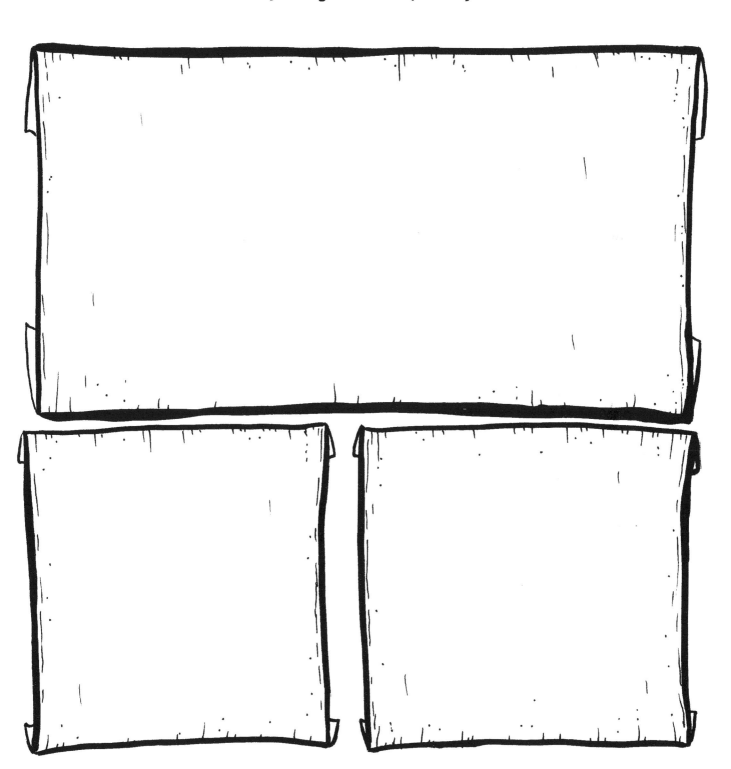

Today's Sport: Volleyball

Date:_____

To-do List:
_____
_____
_____
_____

A Quote:
_____
_____
_____
_____

Today's Moods:

Today's Chores:
_____
_____
_____
_____

Books, Websites & Videos

Resources I can use to study today's sport:

_____
_____
_____

Start your day by watching a competition involving today's sport.

Finish the Story

Bump, set, spike, score! Emma and her Cougar teammates handled the Eagles serve with ease. It was the Cougars serve, and they needed two more points to win the state championships. Emma tossed the ball and served an ace...

_____

_____

_____

_____

_____

_____

_____

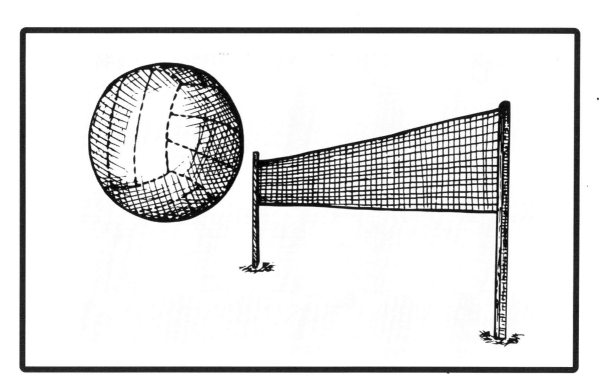

Sports Study

Volleyball

It's research time!

Use the Internet, books, tutorials and documentaries to study this sport. Or go see a game or competition!

Draw any equipment needed for this sport.

Draw a player in uniform.

Draw a trophy or medal for this sport.

Where did this sport originate from?

_____

_____

How was this sport invented?

_____

_____

_____

Who are the main sponsors of the events for this sport?

_____

_____

What is the name of the largest competition where this sport is played? _____

_____

_____

_____

_____

Who is the #1 player of this sport? What makes them the best? How much money do they earn? Where do their earnings come from?

_____

_____

_____

_____

Would you like to play this sport? Why or why not?

_____

_____

What are the common injuries from playing this sport?

_____

_____

_____

Random fact about this sport.

_____

_____

_____

Say What?

Invent your own comic book font and add words to the picture

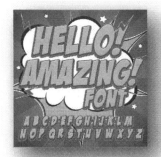
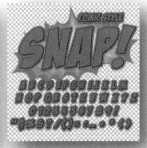
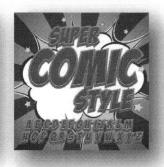
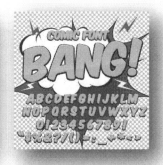

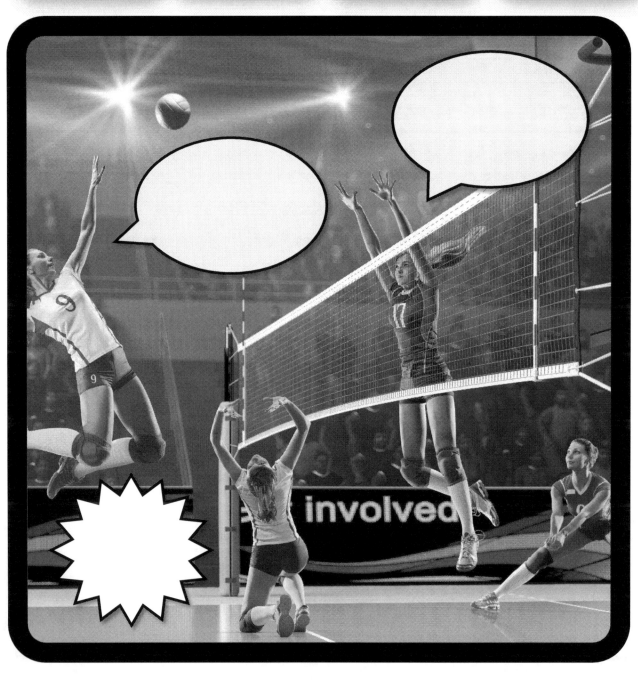

Sports News

Open a newspaper or look online!

What is happening in the world of sports today?

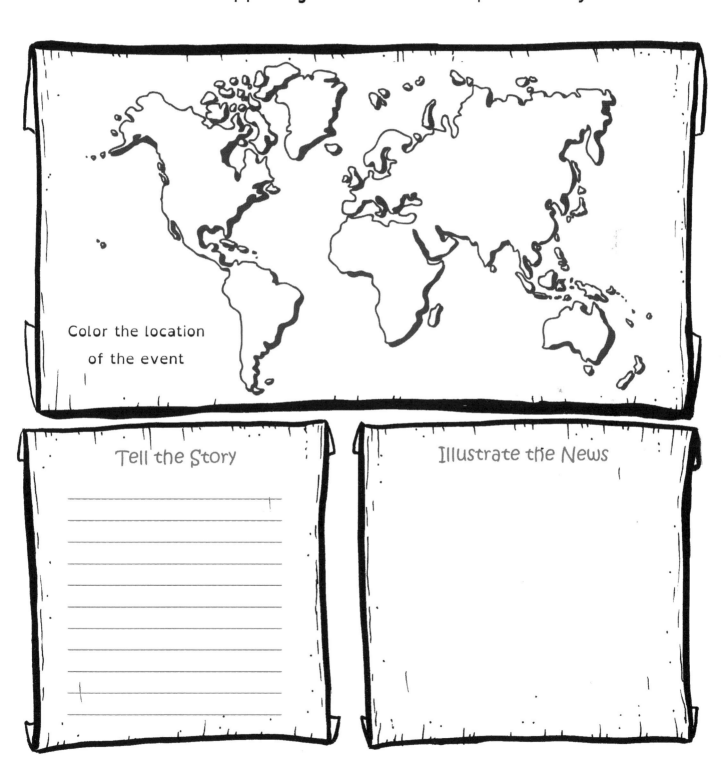

Color the location of the event

Tell the Story

Illustrate the News

Screen Time

Watch a high-quality film, video, tutorial or sports documentary.

Title_____

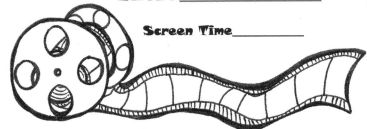

Screen Time_____

Producer_____

Actors_____

_____

_____

_____

Quotes

Draw a scene from the video.

Rating:

worst

Bad

Awful

Ok

Nice

Great

Best

Make a Comic

From the video or your imagination.

Title_____

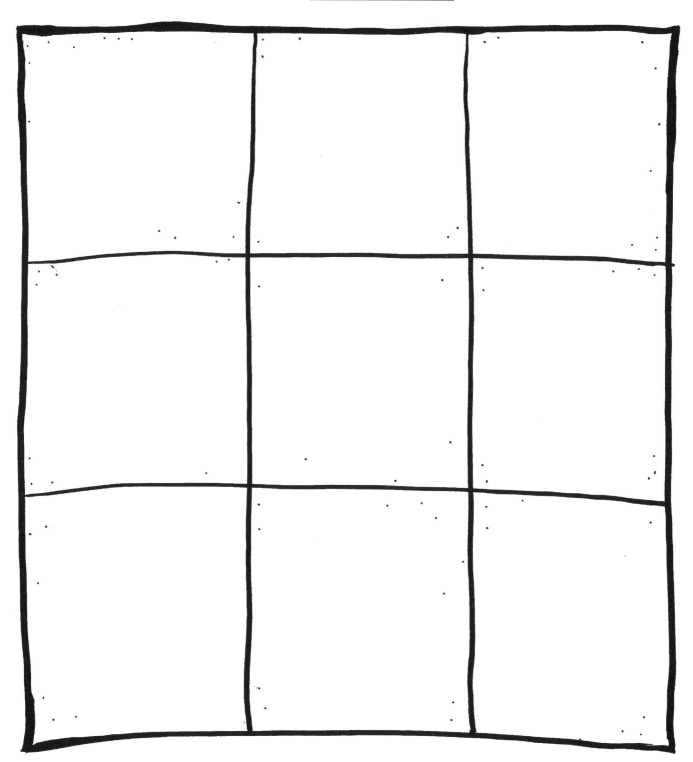

Drawing & Reading Time!

Choose a few books from your stack to focus on today.

Write down and draw anything that inspires you.

(Set a timer for 1 hour)

Free time!

Set the timer for 30 minutes and go outside to play, explore and practice a sport.

What do you plan to do on your free time?

What do you want to practice?

Do you have any goals?

Draw your goals!

Math Practice

Use this page for math practice,

or design a sport's field, rink or play zone

for the sport you are studying today!

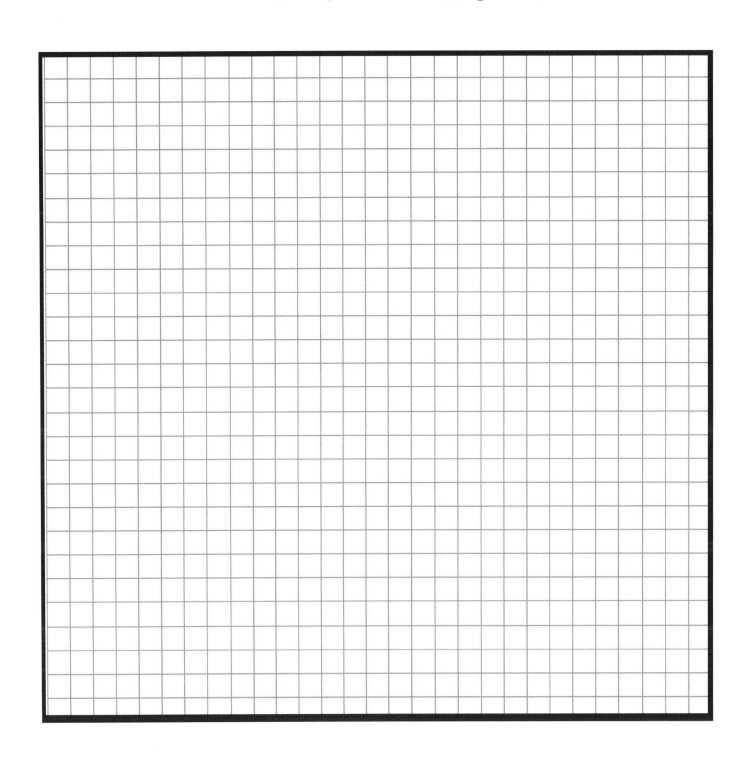

Nature Study

Take this book outside and draw anything and everything that inspires you.

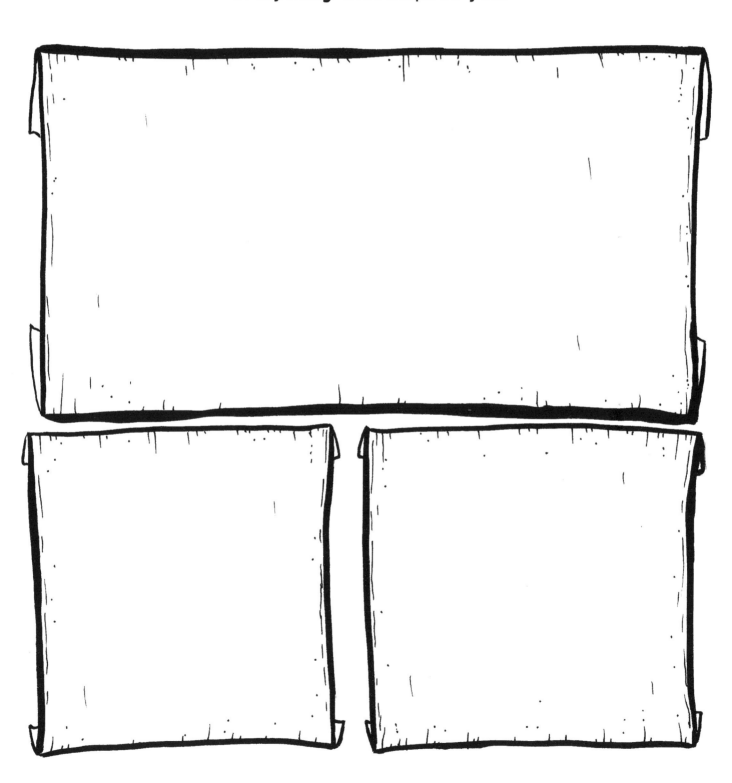

Today's Sport: Cheerleading

Date:_____

To-do List:

_____

_____

_____

_____

A Quote:

_____

_____

_____

_____

Today's Moods:

Today's Chores:

_____

_____

_____

_____

Books, Websites & Videos

Resources I can use to study today's sport:

_____

_____

Start your day by watching a competition involving today's sport.

Math & Research Challenge

Stunts, pyramids, and tosses make up 29.9% of the Hawks total score for the competition. They averaged an 8.2 score for the other 70.1% of the competition. In order to win, they need at least an 8.5 total score. What is the average score they need to earn for stunts, pyramids, and tosses?

Solve the challenge:

_____

_____

_____

_____

_____

_____

ANSWER:

_____

Illustrate your answer:

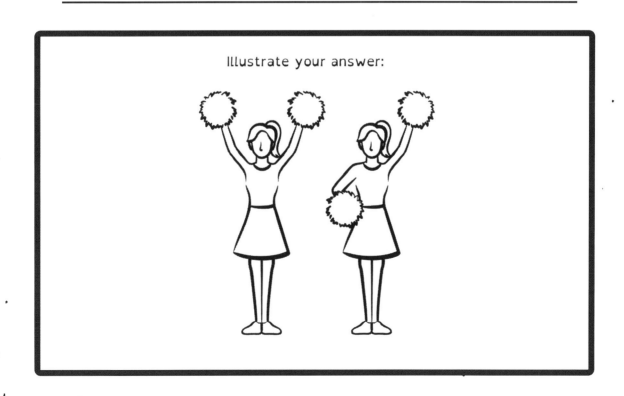

Cheerleading

It's research time!

Use the Internet, books, tutorials and documentaries to study this sport. Or go see a game or competition!

Draw any equipment needed for this sport.

Draw a player in uniform.

Draw a trophy or medal for this sport.

Where did this sport originate from?

_____

_____

How was this sport invented?

_____

_____

_____

Who are the main sponsors of the events for this sport?

_____

_____

What is the name of the largest competition where this sport is played? _____

_____

_____

_____

_____

Who is the #1 player of this sport? What makes them the best? How much money do they earn? Where do their earnings come from?

_____

_____

_____

_____

Would you like to play this sport? Why or why not?

_____

_____

What are the common injuries from playing this sport?

_____

_____

_____

Random fact about this sport.

_____

_____

_____

Say What?

Invent your own comic book font and add words to the picture

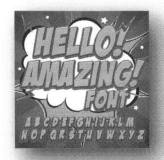
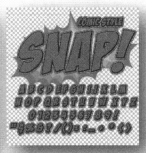
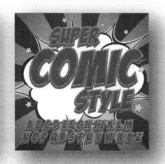
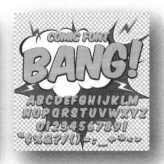

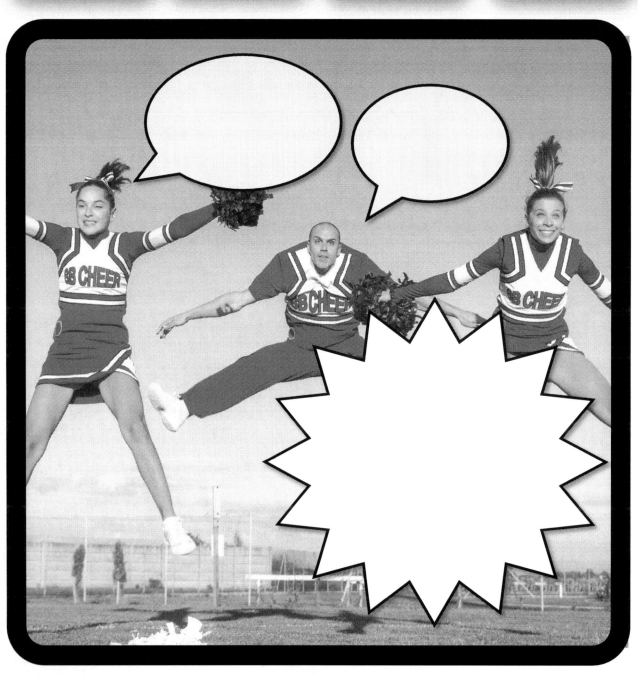

Sports News

Open a newspaper or look online!

What is happening in the world of sports today?

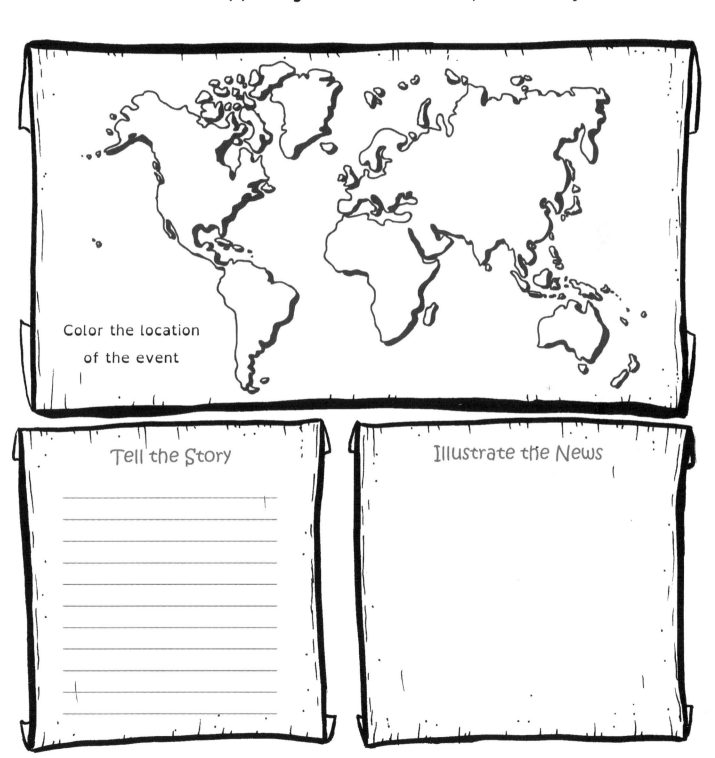

Color the location
of the event

Tell the Story

Illustrate the News

Screen Time

Watch a high-quality film, video, tutorial or sports documentary.

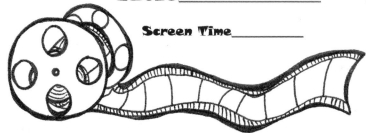

Title_____

Screen Time_____

Producer_____

Actors_____

_____

_____

_____

Quotes

Draw a scene from the video.

Rating:

worst

Bad

Awful

Ok

Nice

Great

Best

Make a Comic

From the video or your imagination.

Title_____

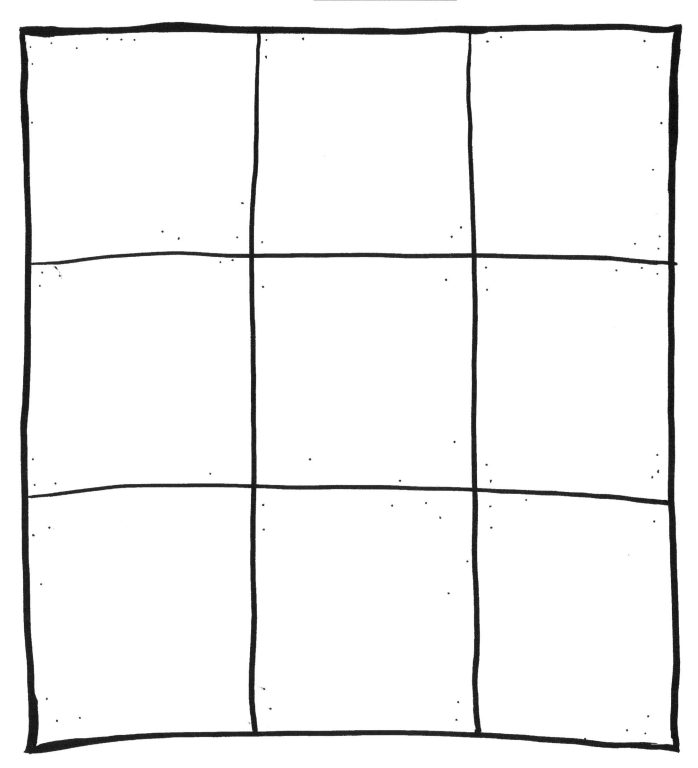

Drawing & Reading Time!

Choose a few books from your stack to focus on today.

Write down and draw anything that inspires you.

(Set a timer for 1 hour)

Free time!

Set the timer for 30 minutes and go outside to play,
explore and practice a sport.

What do you plan to do on your free time?

What do you want to practice?

Do you have any goals?

Draw your goals!

Math Practice

Use this page for math practice,
or design a sport's field, rink or play zone
for the sport you are studying today!

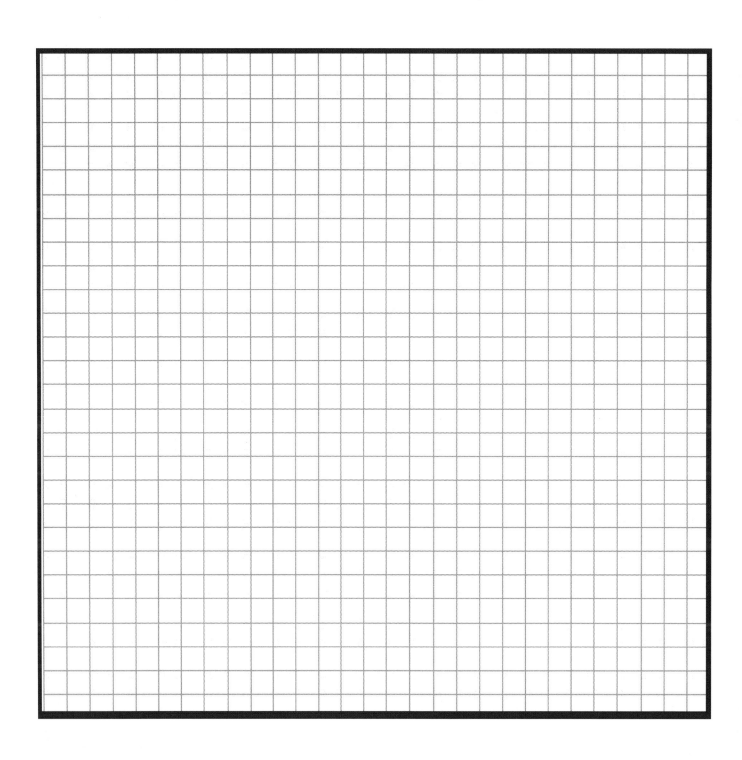

Nature Study

Take this book outside and draw anything and everything that inspires you.

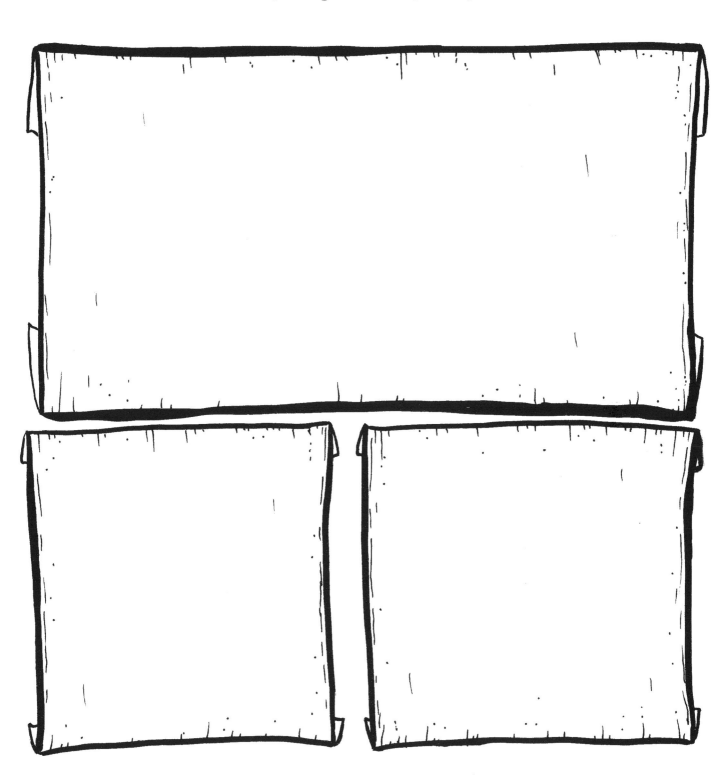

Today's Sport: Archery

Date:_____

To-do List:

_____
_____
_____
_____

A Quote:

_____
_____
_____
_____

Today's Moods:

Today's Chores:

_____
_____
_____
_____

Books, Websites & Videos

Resources I can use to study today's sport:

_____
_____
_____

Start your day by watching a competition involving today's sport.

Math & Research Challenge

In Olympic competitions, archers shoot 72 arrows. Mark the following score: ten points five times, nine points eleven times, eight points eighteen times, seven points fourteen times, six points fifteen times, five points five times, four points twice, three points once, and two points once. What was his total score? What was his average shot score?

Solve the challenge:

_____
_____
_____
_____
_____
_____

ANSWER:

_____

Illustrate your answer:

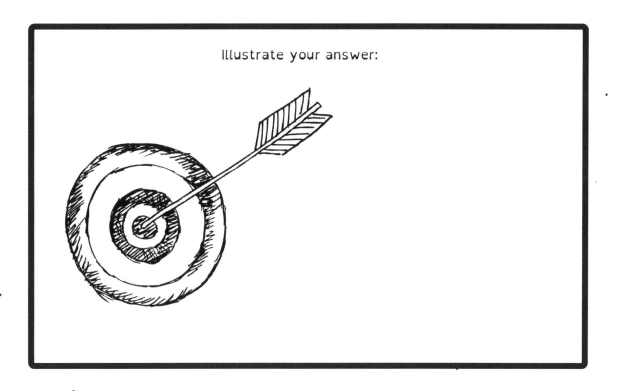

Sports Study

Archery

It's research time!

Use the Internet, books, tutorials and documentaries to study this sport. Or go see a game or competition!

Draw any equipment needed for this sport.

Draw a player in uniform.

Draw a trophy or medal for this sport.

Where did this sport originate from?

_____

_____

How was this sport invented?

_____

_____

_____

Who are the main sponsors of the events for this sport?

_____

_____

What is the name of the largest competition where this sport is played? _____

_____

_____

_____

_____

Who is the #1 player of this sport? What makes them the best? How much money do they earn? Where do their earnings come from?

_____

_____

_____

_____

Would you like to play this sport? Why or why not?

_____

_____

What are the common injuries from playing this sport?

_____

_____

_____

_____

Random fact about this sport.

_____

_____

_____

Say What?

Invent your own comic book font and add words to the picture

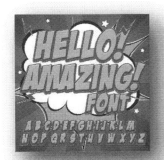
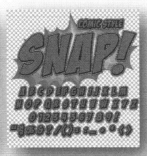
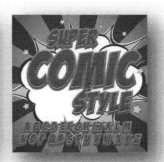
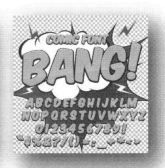

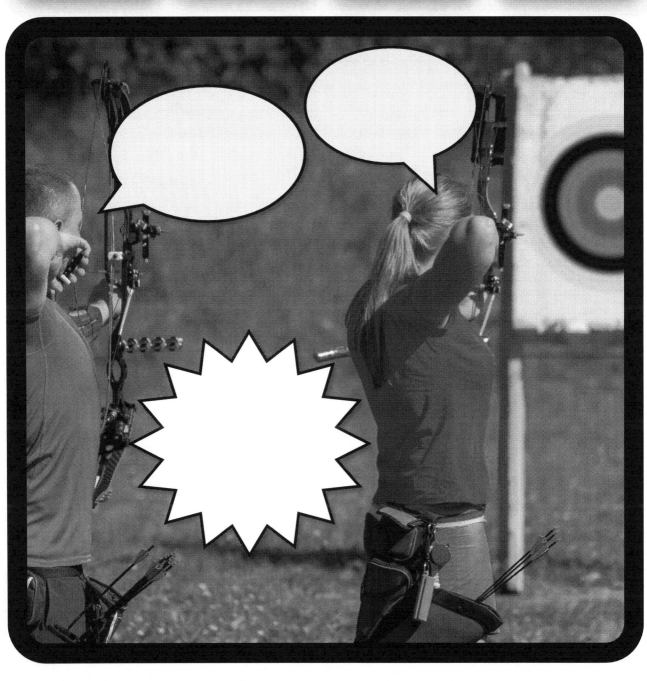

Sports News

Open a newspaper or look online!

What is happening in the world of sports today?

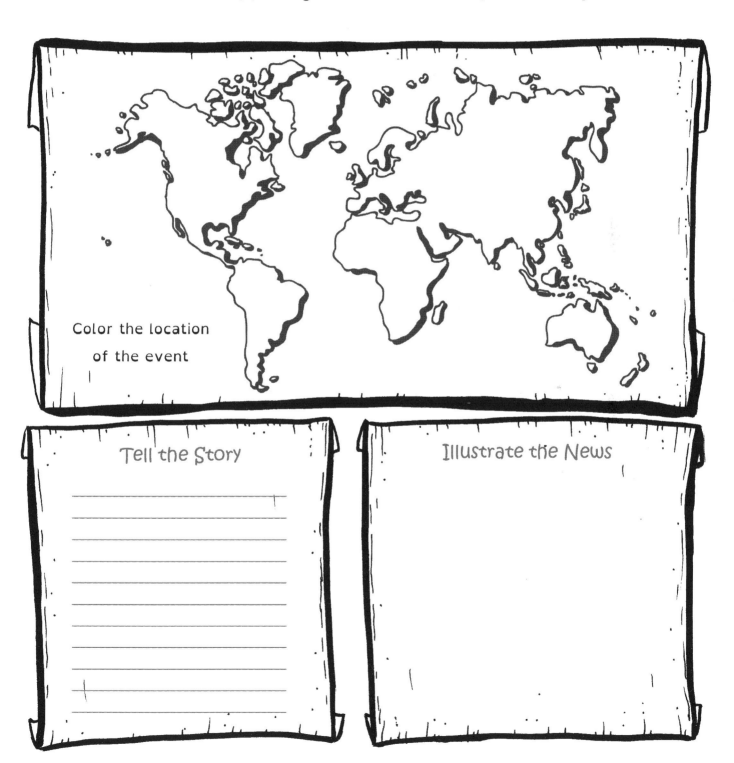

Color the location
of the event

Tell the Story

Illustrate the News

Screen Time

Watch a high-quality film, video, tutorial or sports documentary.

Title_____

Screen Time_____

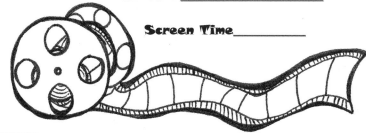

Producer_____

Actors_____

_____

_____

_____

Quotes

Draw a scene from the video.

Rating:

worst

Bad

Awful

Ok

Nice

Great

Best

Make a Comic

From the video or your imagination.

Title_____

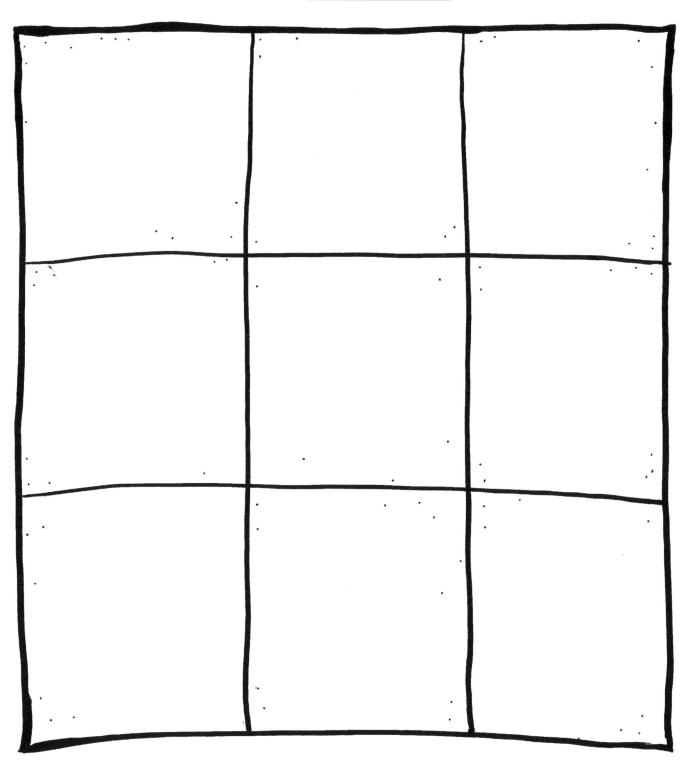

Drawing & Reading Time!

Choose a few books from your stack to focus on today.

Write down and draw anything that inspires you.

(Set a timer for 1 hour)

Free time!

Set the timer for 30 minutes and go outside to play, explore and practice a sport.

What do you plan to do on your free time?

_____

_____

What do you want to practice?

_____

_____

Do you have any goals?

_____

_____

Draw your goals!

Math Practice

Use this page for math practice,

or design a sport's field, rink or play zone

for the sport you are studying today!

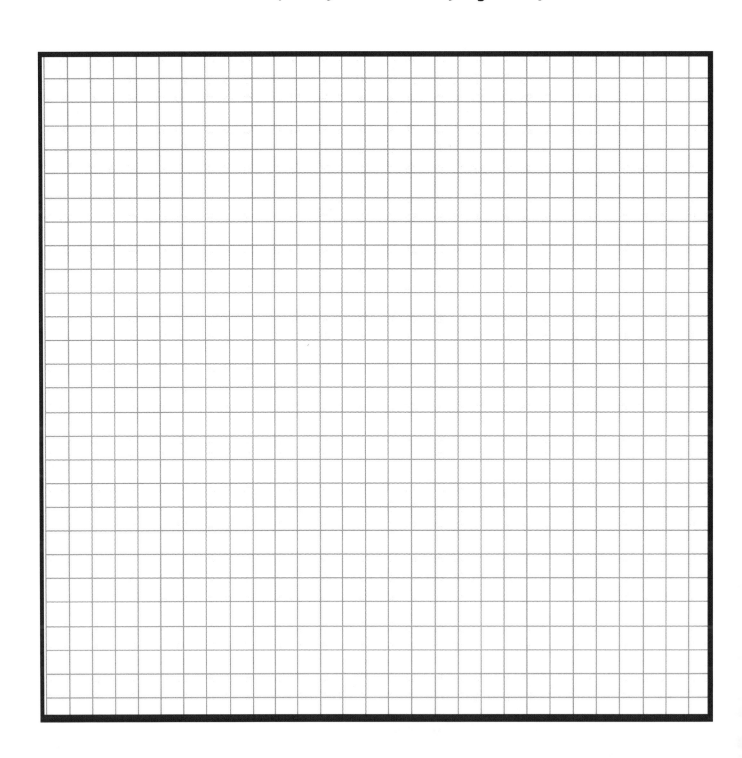

Nature Study

Take this book outside and draw anything and
everything that inspires you.

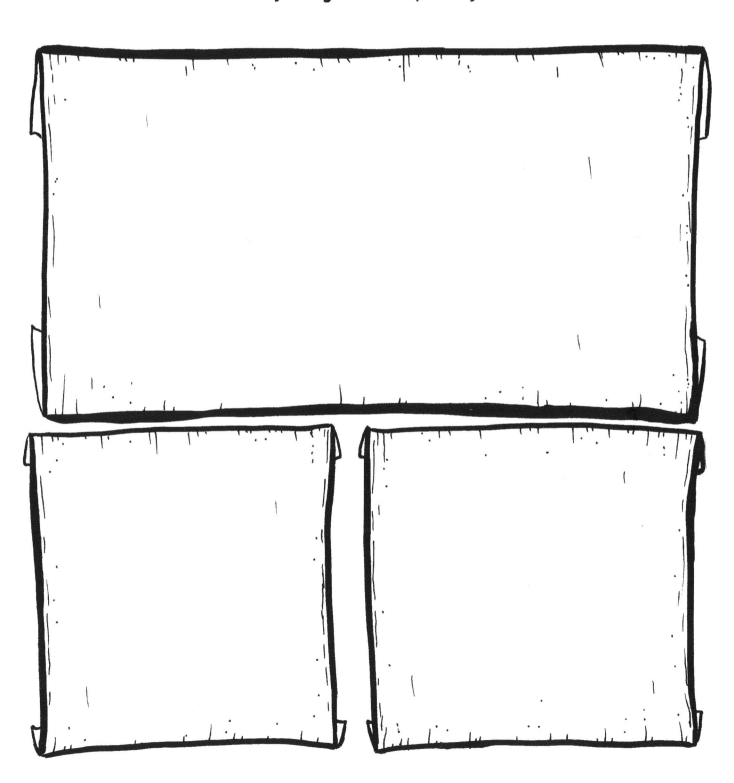

Today's Sport: Snow Skiing

Date:_____

To-do List:
_____
_____
_____
_____
_____

A Quote:
_____
_____
_____
_____
_____

Today's Moods:

Today's Chores:
_____
_____
_____
_____

Books, Websites & Videos

Resources I can use to study today's sport:

_____

_____

_____

Start your day by watching a competition involving today's sport.

Finish the Story

Bentley was at the top of the mountain. He had waited all summer for the first snowfall because this was going to be the year when all his skiing dreams come true. All of a sudden, he heard this horrible crushing noise beneath him. The ground started shaking...

_____

_____

_____

_____

_____

_____

_____

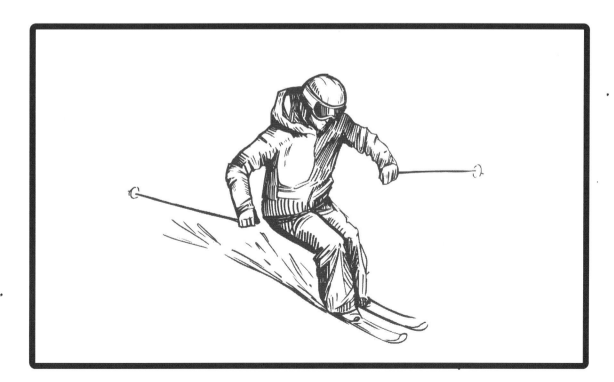

Snow Skiing

It's research time!

Use the Internet, books, tutorials and documentaries to study
this sport. Or go see a game or competition!

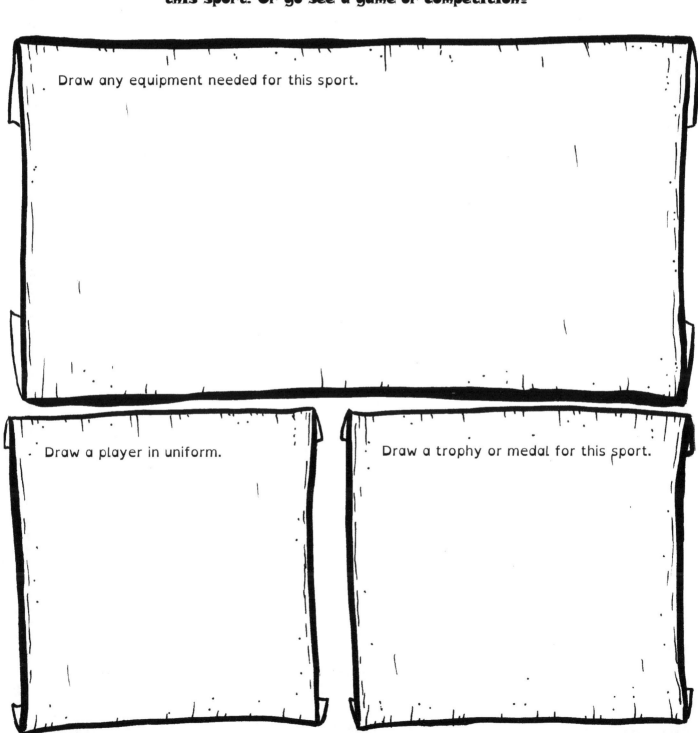

Draw any equipment needed for this sport.

Draw a player in uniform.

Draw a trophy or medal for this sport.

Where did this sport originate from?

_____

_____

How was this sport invented?

_____

_____

_____

Who are the main sponsors of the events for this sport?

_____

_____

What is the name of the largest competition where this sport is played? _____

_____

_____

_____

_____

Who is the #1 player of this sport? What makes them the best? How much money do they earn? Where do their earnings come from?

_____

_____

_____

_____

Would you like to play this sport? Why or why not?

_____

_____

What are the common injuries from playing this sport?

_____

_____

_____

Random fact about this sport.

_____

_____

_____

Say What?

Invent your own comic book font and add words to the picture

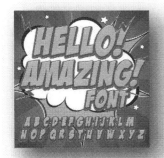
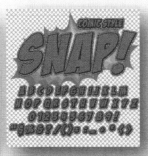
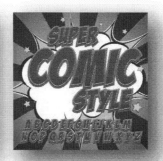
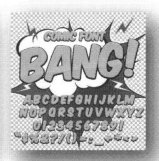

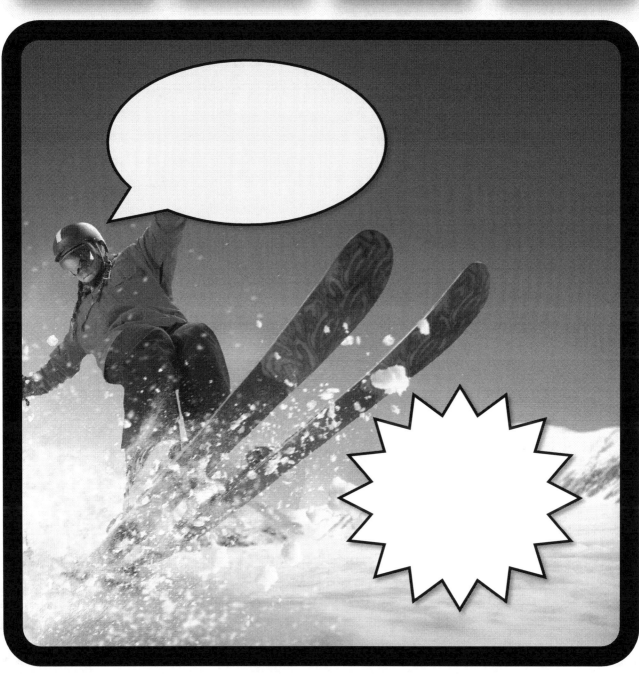

Sports News

Open a newspaper or look online!

What is happening in the world of sports today?

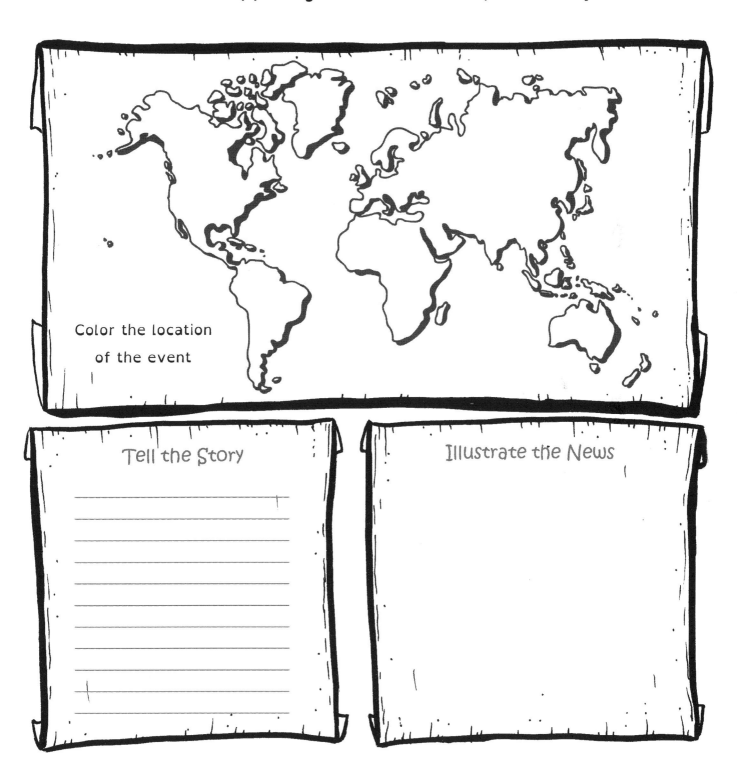

Color the location
of the event

Tell the Story

Illustrate the News

Screen Time

Watch a high-quality film, video, tutorial or sports documentary.

Title_____

Screen Time_____

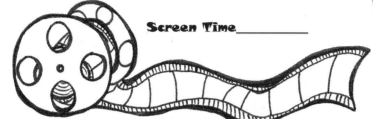

Producer_____

Actors_____

_____

_____

_____

Quotes

Draw a scene from the video.

Rating:

worst

Bad

Awful

Ok

Nice

Great

Best

Make a Comic

From the video or your imagination.

Title_____

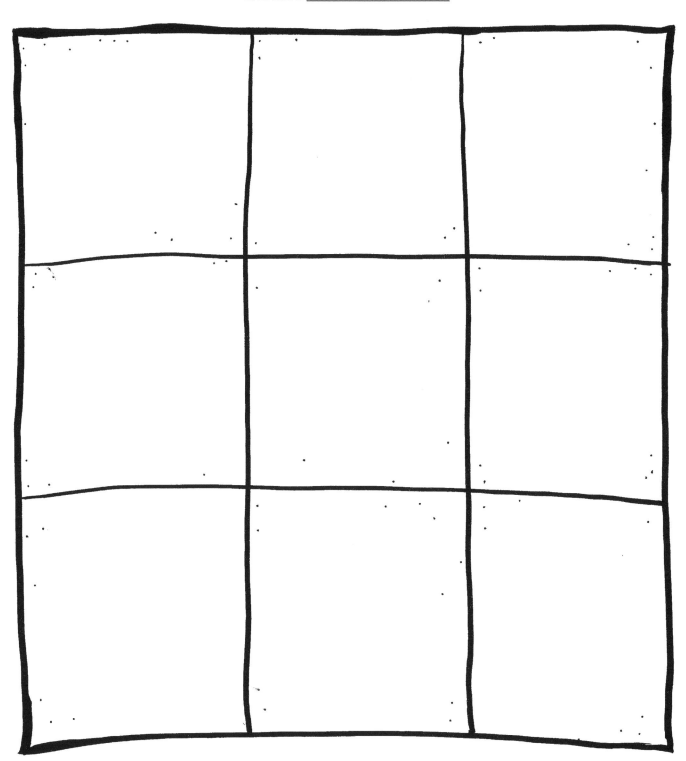

Drawing & Reading Time!

Choose a few books from your stack to focus on today.

Write down and draw anything that inspires you.

(Set a timer for 1 hour)

Free time!

Set the timer for 30 minutes and go outside to play, explore and practice a sport.

What do you plan to do on your free time?

What do you want to practice?

Do you have any goals?

Draw your goals!

Math Practice

Use this page for math practice,

or design a sport's field, rink or play zone

for the sport you are studying today!

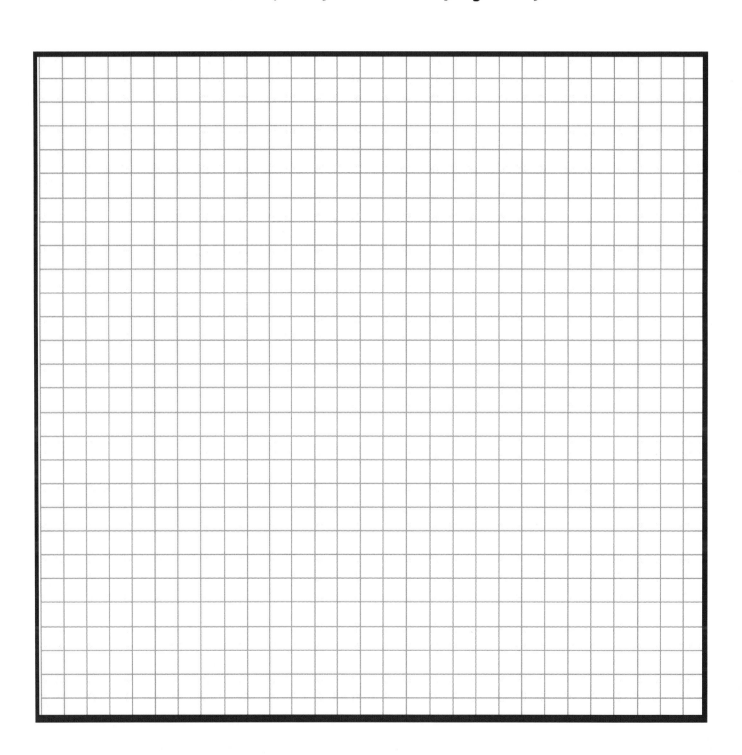

Nature Study

Take this book outside and draw anything and everything that inspires you.

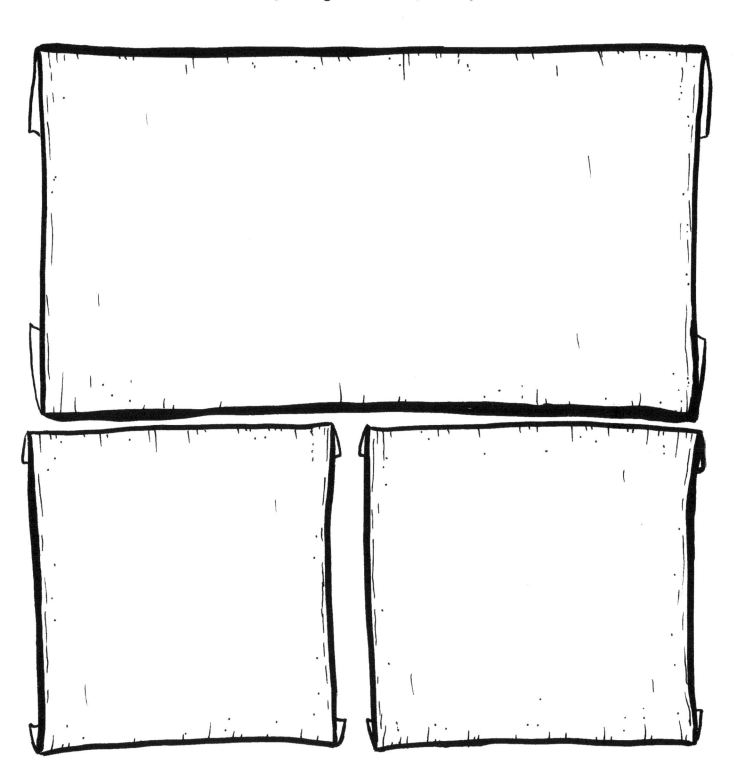

Today's Sport: Martial Arts

Date:_____

To-do List:
_____
_____
_____
_____
_____

A Quote:
_____
_____
_____
_____

Today's Moods:

Today's Chores:
_____
_____
_____
_____

Books, Websites & Videos

Resources I can use to study today's sport:

_____
_____
_____

Start your day by watching a competition involving today's sport.

Math & Research Challenge

In order to advance to the next belt, Gabriel has to attend an hour-long class twice a week for 14 weeks and practice for an additional 4 hours per week. At the end of the 14 weeks, how many hours will Gabriel have worked on his martial arts between his class and practice?

Solve the challenge:

_____
_____
_____
_____
_____
_____

ANSWER:

_____

Illustrate your answer:

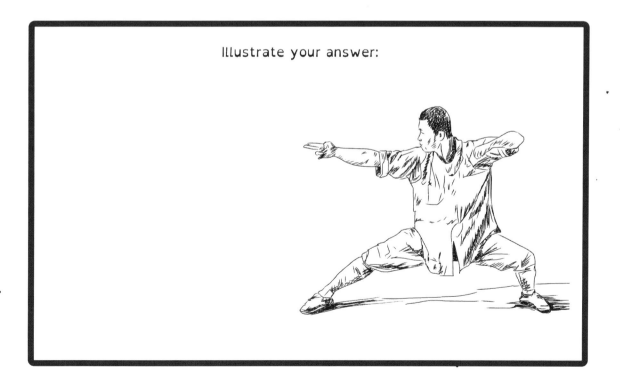

Martial Arts

It's research time!

Use the Internet, books, tutorials and documentaries to study
this sport. Or go see a game or competition!

Draw any equipment needed for this sport.

Draw a player in uniform.

Draw a trophy or medal for this sport.

Where did this sport originate from?

_____

_____

How was this sport invented?

_____

_____

_____

Who are the main sponsors of the events for this sport?

_____

_____

What is the name of the largest competition where this sport is played? _____

_____

_____

_____

_____

Who is the #1 player of this sport? What makes them the best? How much money do they earn? Where do their earnings come from?

_____

_____

_____

_____

Would you like to play this sport? Why or why not?

_____

_____

What are the common injuries from playing this sport?

_____

_____

_____

Random fact about this sport.

_____

_____

_____

Say What?

Invent your own comic book font and add words to the picture

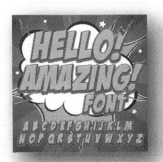
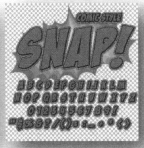
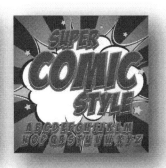
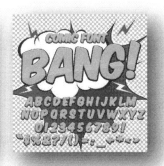

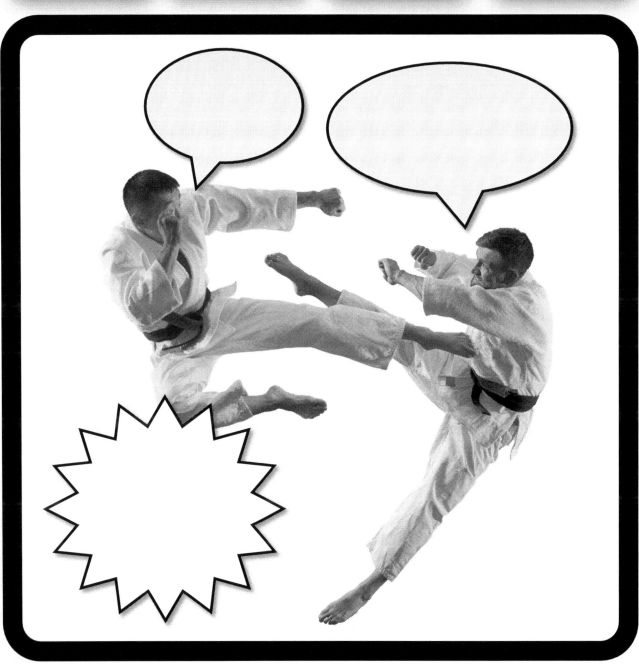

Sports News

Open a newspaper or look online!

What is happening in the world of sports today?

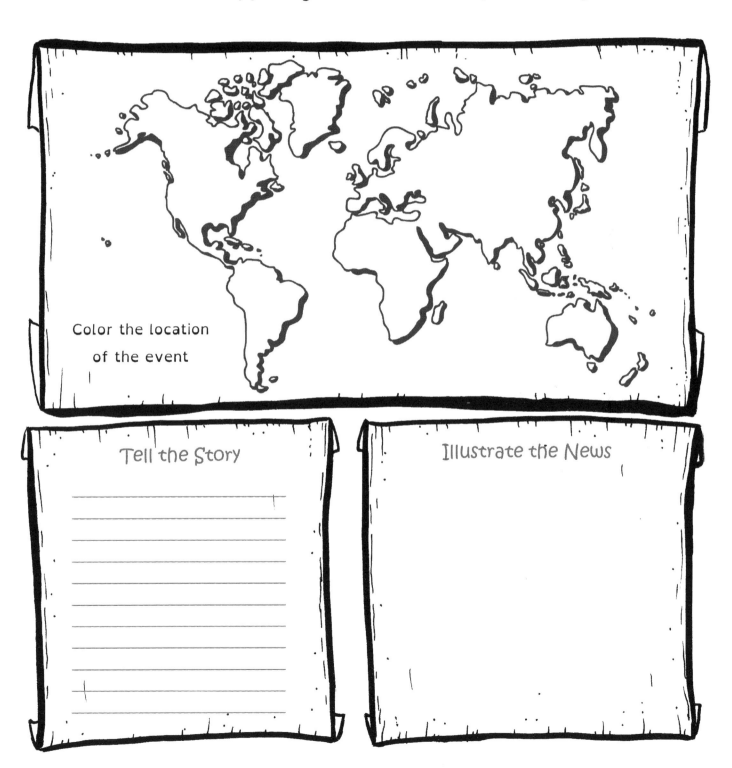

Color the location
of the event

Tell the Story

Illustrate the News

Screen Time

Watch a high-quality film, video, tutorial or sports documentary.

Title_____

Screen Time_____

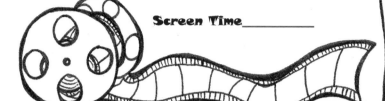

Producer_____

Actors_____

_____

_____

_____

Quotes

Draw a scene from the video.

Rating:

worst

Bad

Awful

Ok

Nice

Great

Best

Make a Comic

From the video or your imagination.

Title_____

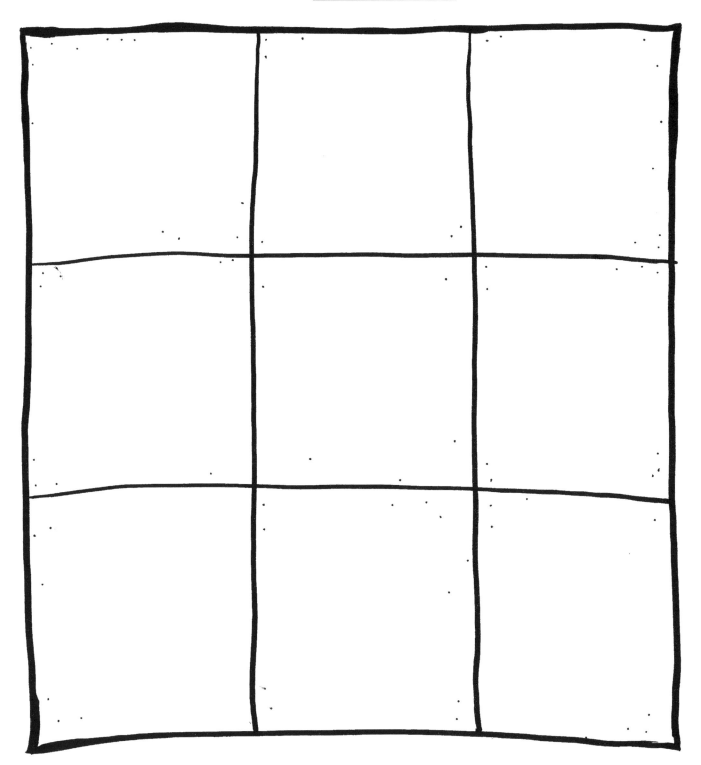

Drawing & Reading Time!

Choose a few books from your stack to focus on today.

Write down and draw anything that inspires you.

(Set a timer for 1 hour)

Free time!

Set the timer for 30 minutes and go outside to play, explore and practice a sport.

What do you plan to do on your free time?

_____

_____

What do you want to practice?

_____

_____

Do you have any goals?

_____

_____

Draw your goals!

Math Practice

Use this page for math practice,

or design a sport's field, rink or play zone

for the sport you are studying today!

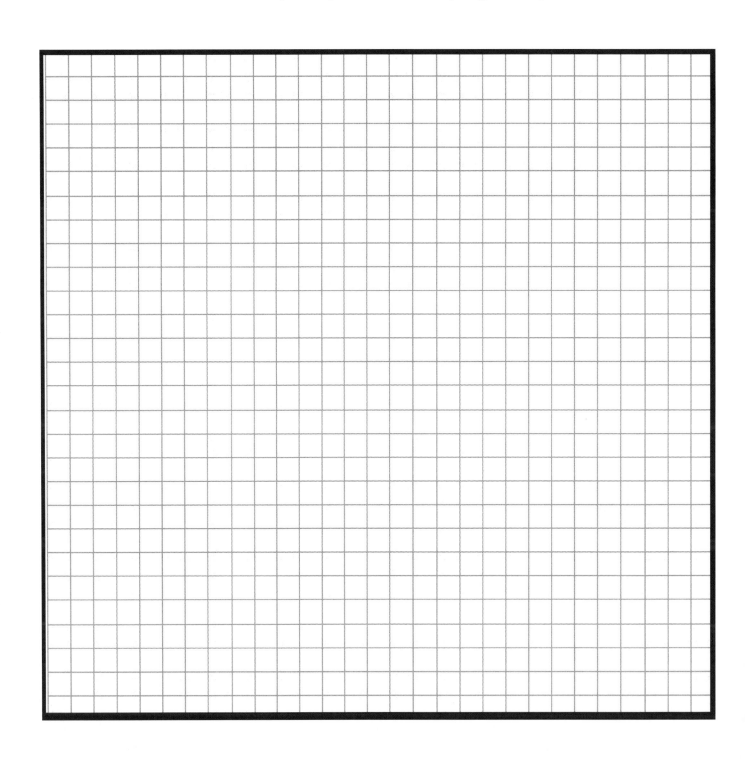

Nature Study

Take this book outside and draw anything and
everything that inspires you.

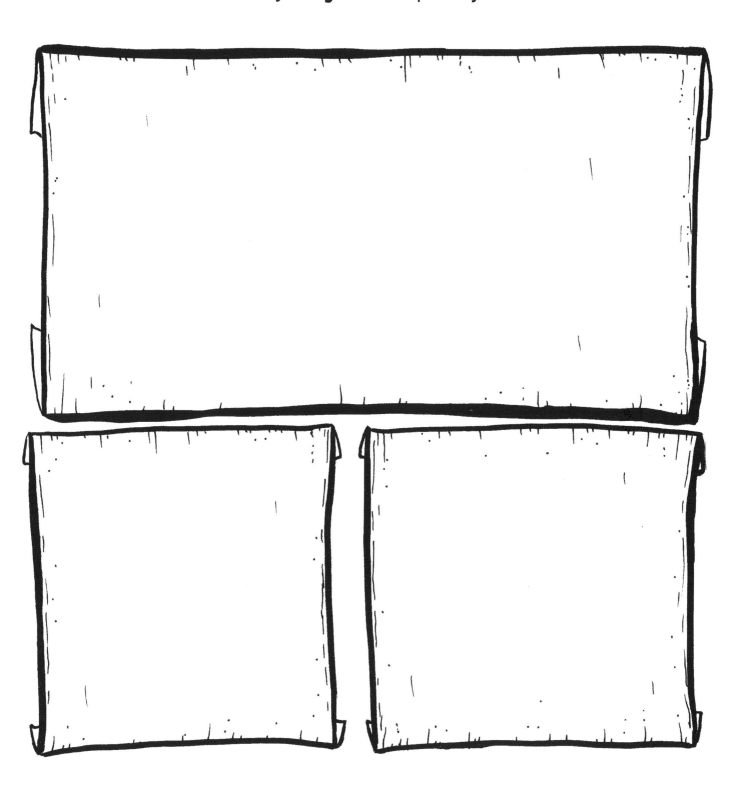

Today's Sport: Hunting

Date:_____

To-do List:

_____

_____

_____

_____

A Quote:

_____

_____

_____

_____

Today's Moods:

Today's Chores:

_____

_____

_____

_____

Books, Websites & Videos

Resources I can use to study today's sport:

_____

_____

_____

Start your day by watching a competition involving today's sport.

Finish the Story

David is an avid hunter and has recently moved to the mountains of Tennessee. Before going hunting he begins to research the hunting laws in his state.

He is surprised that some of the hunting regulations will limit his plans. What did he discover and what will he do?

_____

_____

_____

_____

_____

_____

_____

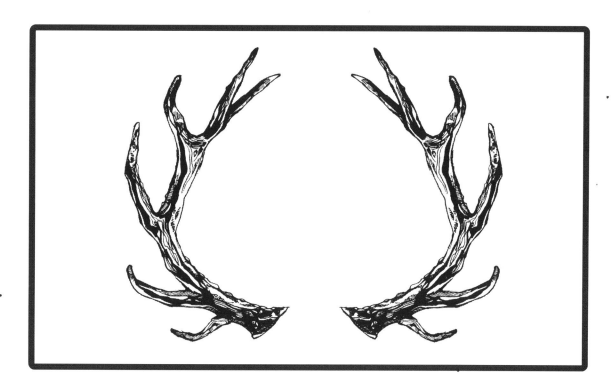

Sports Study

Hunting

It's research time!

Use the Internet, books, tutorials and documentaries to study
this sport. Or go see a game or competition!

Draw any equipment needed for this sport.

Draw a player in uniform.

Draw a trophy or medal for this sport.

Where did this sport originate from?

_____

_____

How was this sport invented?

_____

_____

_____

Who are the main sponsors of the events for this sport?

_____

_____

What is the name of the largest competition where this sport is played? _____

_____

_____

_____

Who is the #1 player of this sport? What makes them the best? How much money do they earn? Where do their earnings come from?

_____

_____

_____

_____

Would you like to play this sport? Why or why not?

_____

_____

What are the common injuries from playing this sport?

_____

_____

_____

Random fact about this sport.

_____

_____

_____

Say What?

Invent your own comic book font and add words to the picture

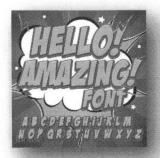
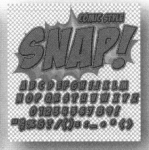
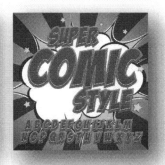
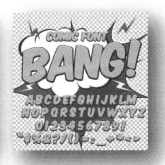

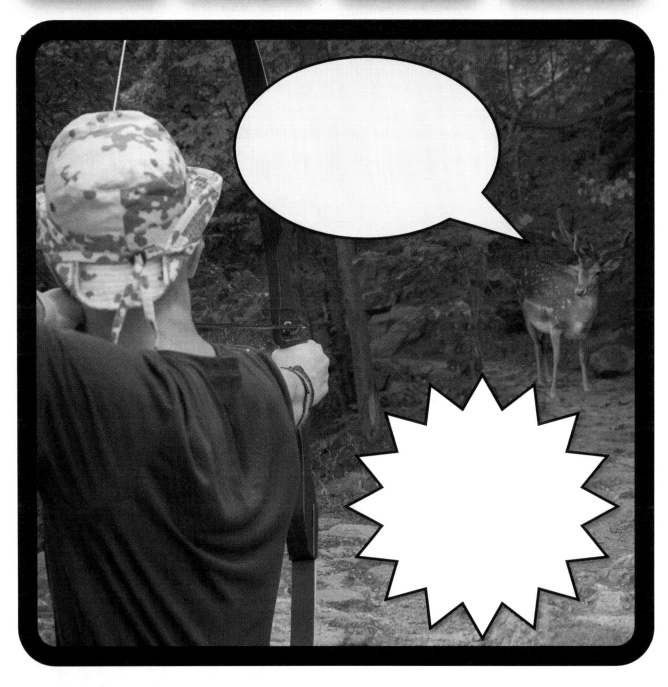

Sports News

Open a newspaper or look online!

What is happening in the world of sports today?

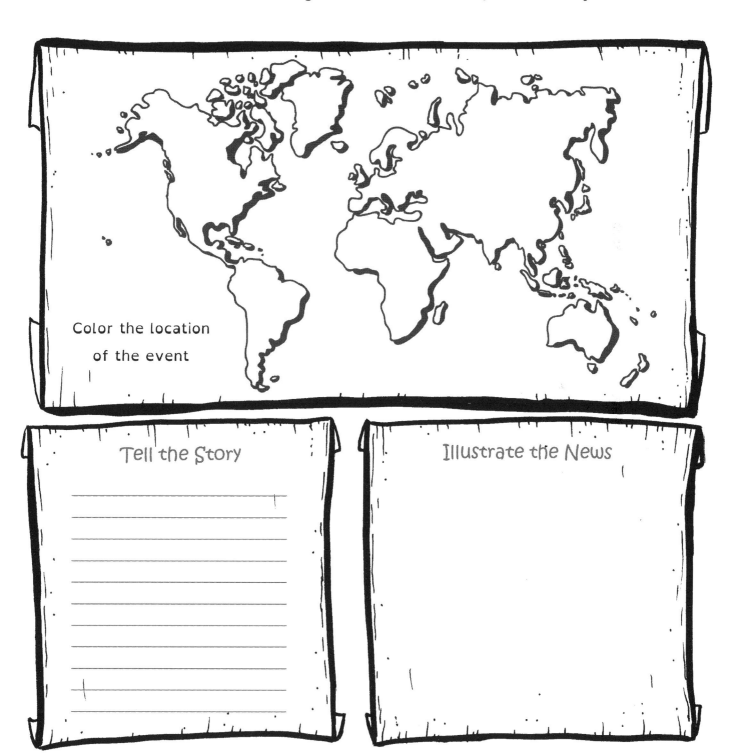

Color the location
of the event

Tell the Story

Illustrate the News

Screen Time

Watch a high-quality film, video, tutorial or sports documentary.

Title_____

Screen Time_____

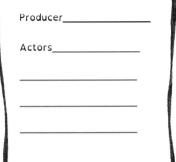

Producer_____

Actors_____

_____

_____

_____

Quotes

Draw a scene from the video.

Rating:

worst

Bad

Awful

Ok

Nice

Great

Best

Make a Comic

From the video or your imagination.

Title_____

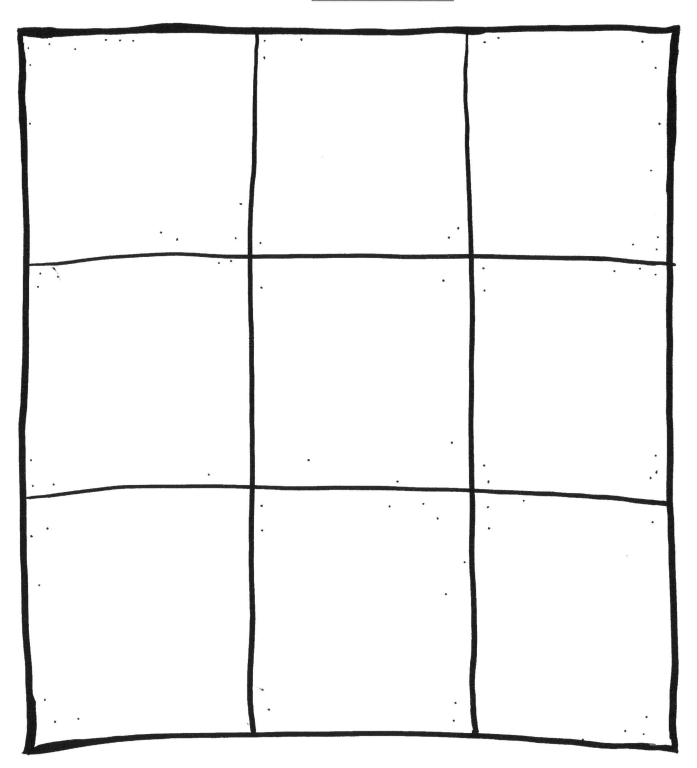

Drawing & Reading Time!

Choose a few books from your stack to focus on today.

Write down and draw anything that inspires you.

(Set a timer for 1 hour)

Free time!

Set the timer for 30 minutes and go outside to play,
explore and practice a sport.

What do you plan to do on your free time?

What do you want to practice?

Do you have any goals?

Draw your goals!

Math Practice

Use this page for math practice,

or design a sport's field, rink or play zone

for the sport you are studying today!

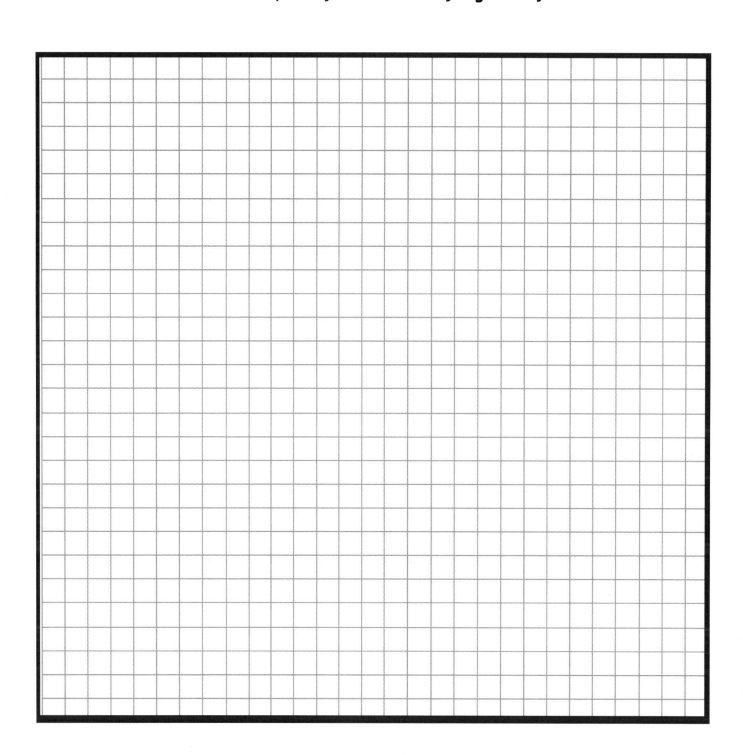

Nature Study

Take this book outside and draw anything and
everything that inspires you.

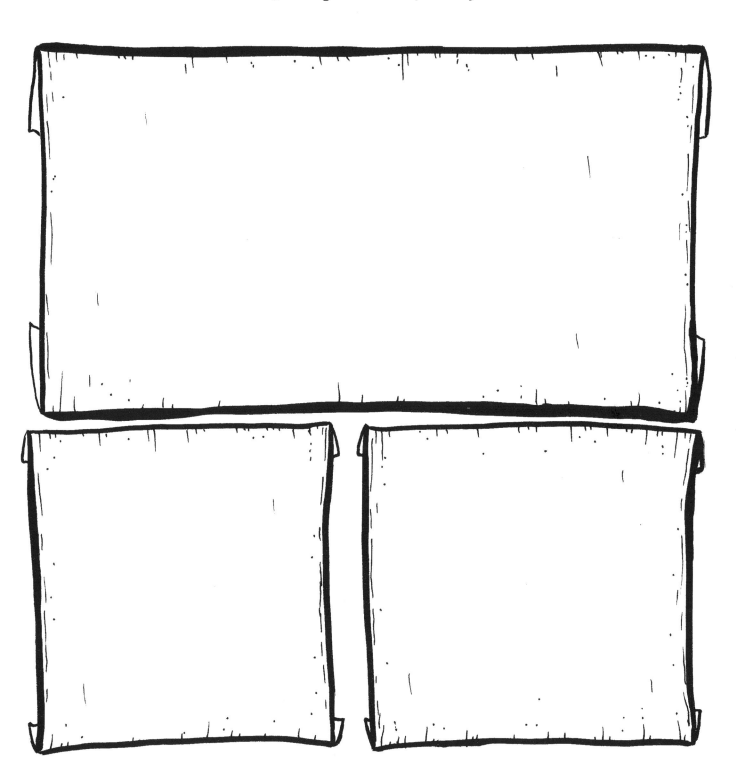

Today's Sport: Figure Skating

Date:_____

To-do List:
_____
_____
_____
_____

A Quote:
_____
_____
_____
_____

Today's Moods:

Today's Chores:
_____
_____
_____
_____

Books, Websites & Videos

Resources I can use to study today's sport:

_____
_____
_____

Start your day by watching a competition involving today's sport.

Finish the Story

Sarah woke up to bright lights in her eyes. As she slowly came to, she began remembering the details of how she came to be here. She had landed that jump so many times before, but the pain in her legs reminded her of her last memories in the rink...

_____
_____
_____
_____
_____
_____
_____

Illustrate your story:

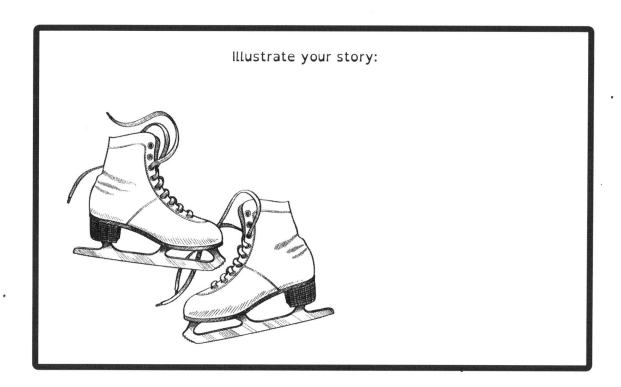

Figure Skating

It's research time!

Use the Internet, books, tutorials and documentaries to study this sport. Or go see a game or competition!

Draw any equipment needed for this sport.

Draw a player in uniform.

Draw a trophy or medal for this sport.

Where did this sport originate from?

_____

_____

How was this sport invented?

_____

_____

_____

Who are the main sponsors of the events for this sport?

_____

_____

What is the name of the largest competition where this sport is played? _____

_____

_____

_____

_____

Who is the #1 player of this sport? What makes them the best? How much money do they earn? Where do their earnings come from?

_____

_____

_____

_____

Would you like to play this sport? Why or why not?

_____

_____

What are the common injuries from playing this sport?

_____

_____

_____

Random fact about this sport.

_____

_____

_____

Say What?

Invent your own comic book font and add words to the picture

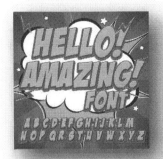
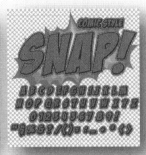
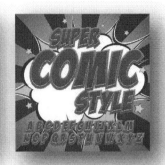
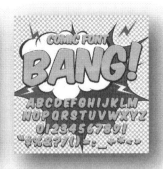

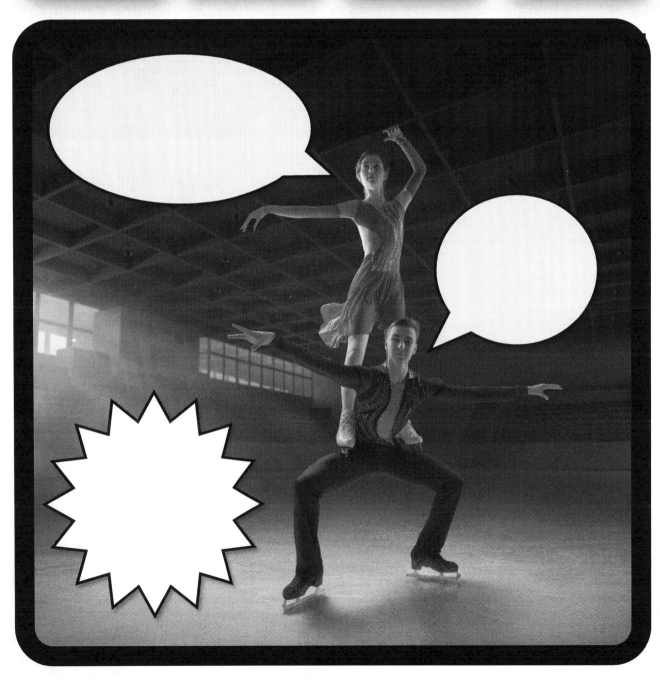

Sports News

Open a newspaper or look online!

What is happening in the world of sports today?

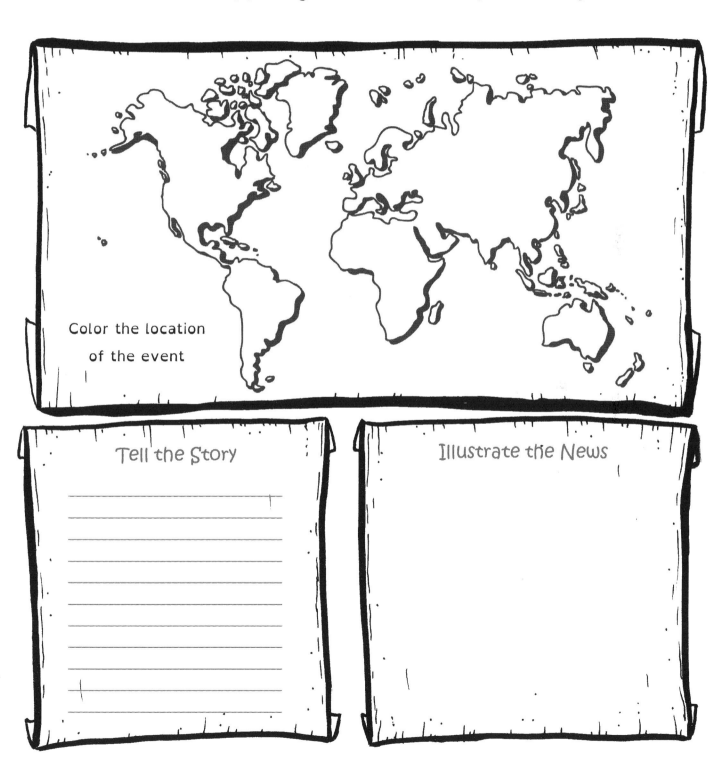

Color the location
of the event

Tell the Story

Illustrate the News

Screen Time

Watch a high-quality film, video, tutorial or sports documentary.

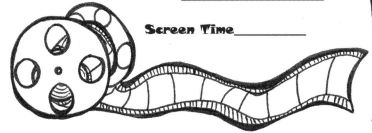

Title_____

Screen Time_____

Producer_____

Actors_____

_____

_____

_____

Quotes

Draw a scene from the video.

Rating:

worst

Bad

Awful

Ok

Nice

Great

Best

Make a Comic

From the video or your imagination.

Title_____

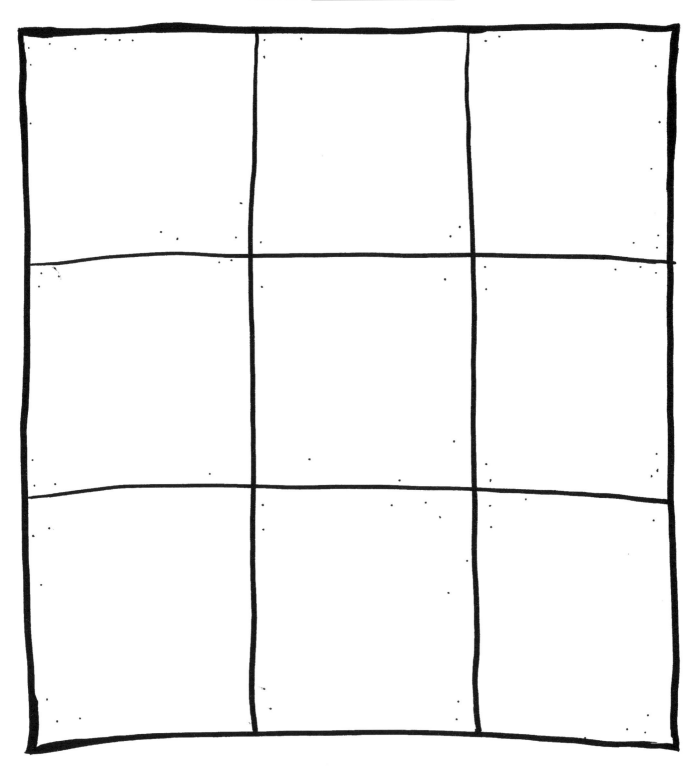

Drawing & Reading Time!

Choose a few books from your stack to focus on today.

Write down and draw anything that inspires you.

(Set a timer for 1 hour)

Free time!

Set the timer for 30 minutes and go outside to play, explore and practice a sport.

What do you plan to do on your free time?

What do you want to practice?

Do you have any goals?

Draw your goals!

Math Practice

Use this page for math practice,

or design a sport's field, rink or play zone

for the sport you are studying today!

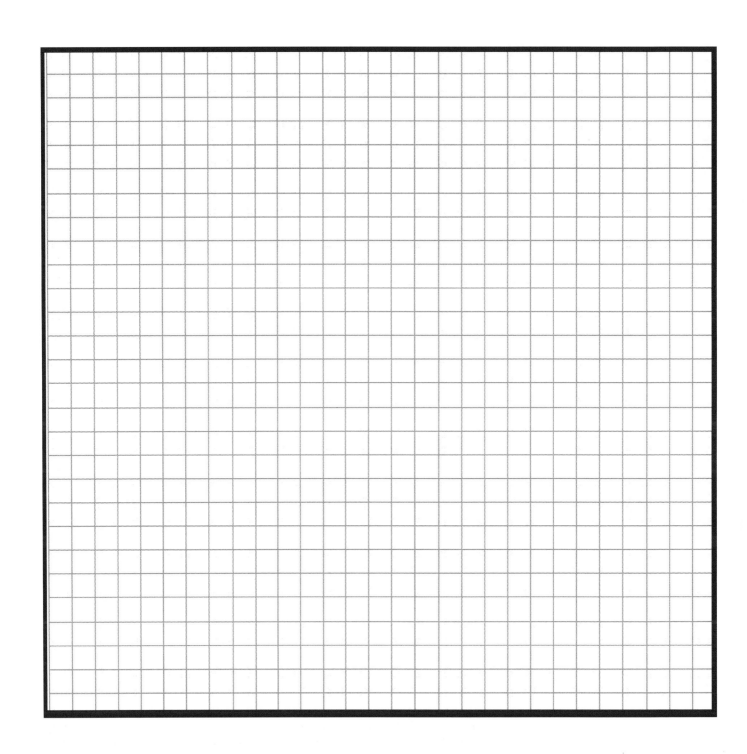

Nature Study

Take this book outside and draw anything and everything that inspires you.

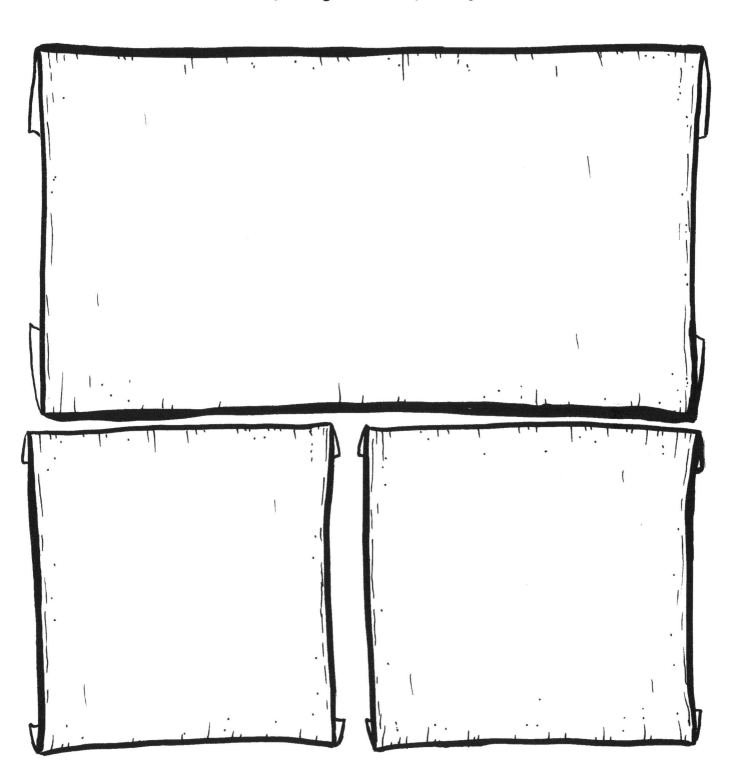

Today's Sport: Chess

Date:_____

To-do List:
_____
_____
_____
_____

A Quote:
_____
_____
_____
_____

Today's Moods:

Today's Chores:
_____
_____
_____
_____

Books, Websites & Videos

Resources I can use to study today's sport:

_____
_____
_____

Start your day by watching a competition involving today's sport.

Math & Research Challenge

In tournaments, players are granted 1 point for a win, 1/2 point for a draw, and 0 points for a loss. Peter won 4, had a draw on 2, and lost 2. Andrew won 3, had a draw on 4, and lost 1. Who won between Peter and Andrew?

Solve the challenge:

_____

_____

_____

_____

_____

_____

ANSWER:

_____

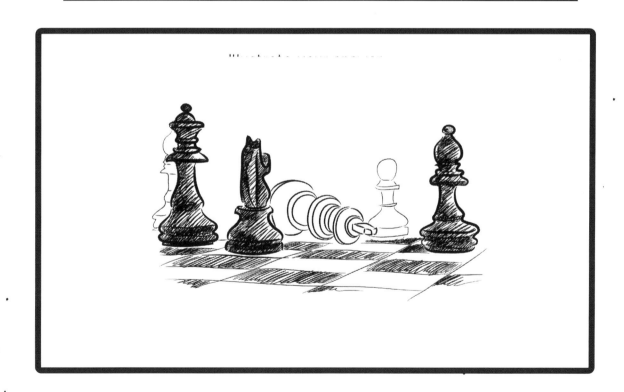

Illustrate your answer

Sports Study

Chess

It's research time!

Use the Internet, books, tutorials and documentaries to study this sport. Or go see a game or competition!

Draw any equipment needed for this sport.

Draw a player in uniform.

Draw a trophy or medal for this sport.

Where did this sport originate from?

_____

_____

How was this sport invented?

_____

_____

_____

Who are the main sponsors of the events for this sport?

_____

_____

What is the name of the largest competition where this sport is played? _____

_____

_____

_____

_____

Who is the #1 player of this sport? What makes them the best? How much money do they earn? Where do their earnings come from?

_____

_____

_____

_____

Would you like to play this sport? Why or why not?

_____

_____

What are the common injuries from playing this sport?

_____

_____

_____

Random fact about this sport.

_____

_____

_____

Say What?

Invent your own comic book font and add words to the picture

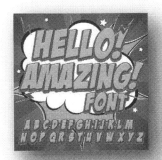
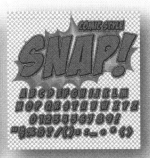
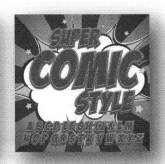
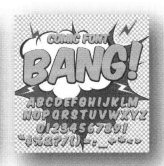

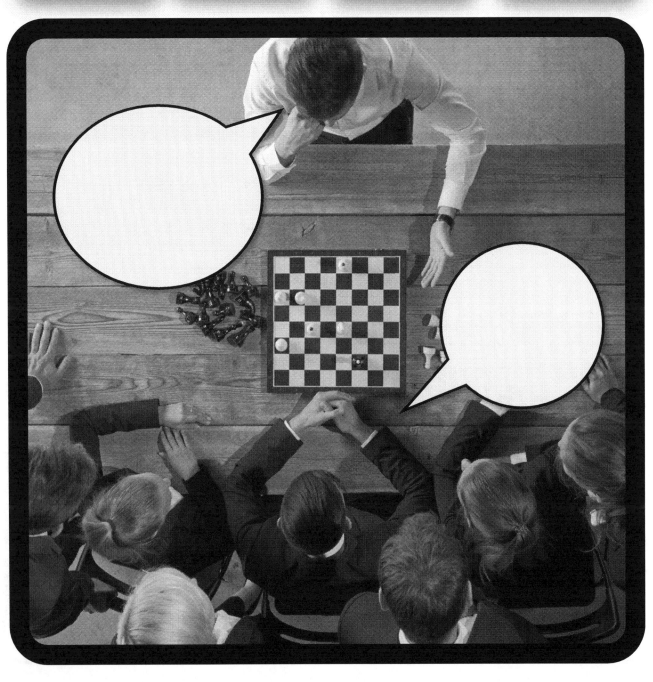

Sports News

Open a newspaper or look online!

What is happening in the world of sports today?

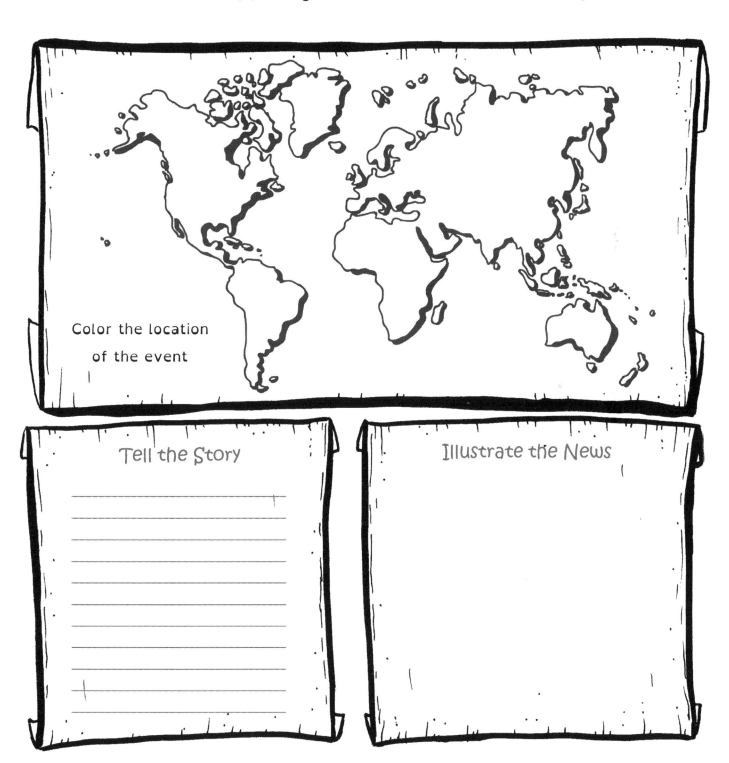

Color the location
of the event

Tell the Story

Illustrate the News

Screen Time

Watch a high-quality film, video, tutorial or sports documentary.

Title_____

Screen Time_____

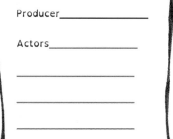

Producer_____

Actors_____

_____

_____

_____

Quotes

Draw a scene from the video.

Rating:

worst

Bad

Awful

Ok

Nice

Great

Best

Make a Comic

From the video or your imagination.

Title _____

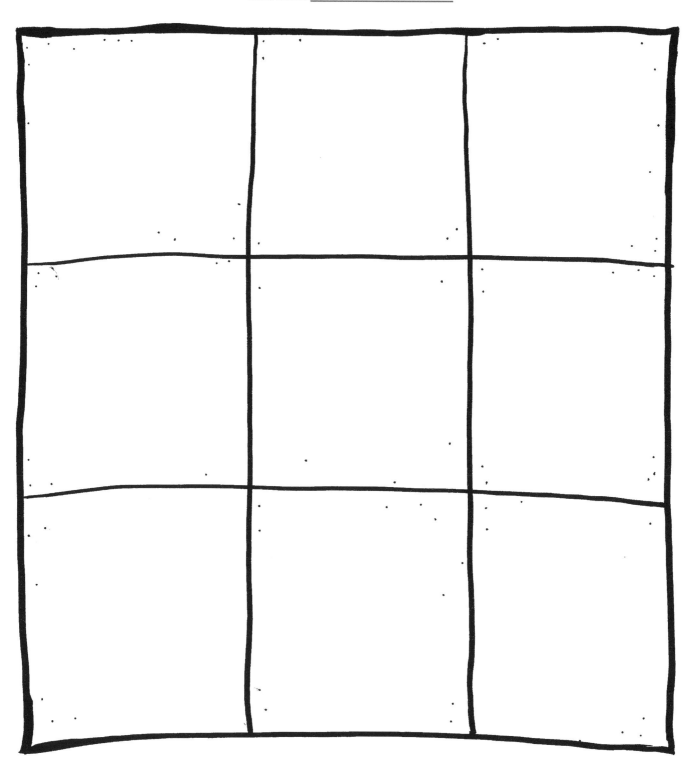

Drawing & Reading Time!

Choose a few books from your stack to focus on today.

Write down and draw anything that inspires you.

(Set a timer for 1 hour)

Free time!

Set the timer for 30 minutes and go outside to play, explore and practice a sport.

What do you plan to do on your free time?

_____

_____

What do you want to practice?

_____

_____

Do you have any goals?

_____

_____

Draw your goals!

Math Practice

Use this page for math practice,

or design a sport's field, rink or play zone

for the sport you are studying today!

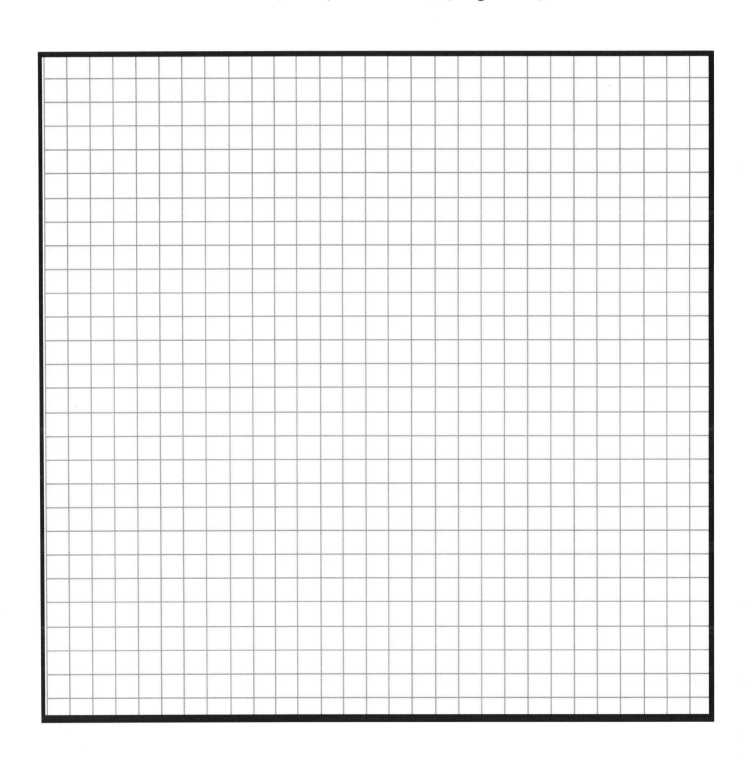

Nature Study

Take this book outside and draw anything and everything that inspires you.

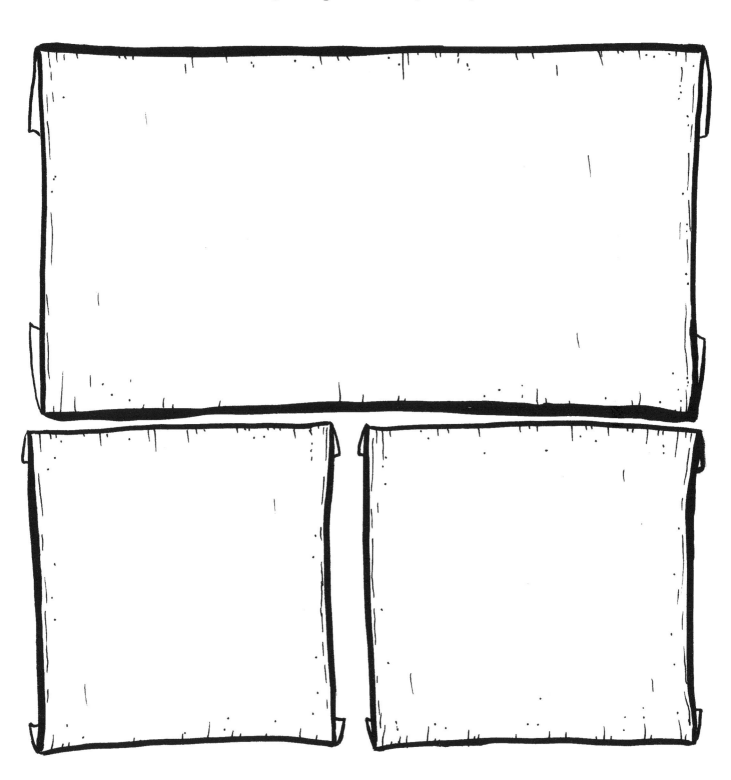

Today's Sport: Kayaking

Date:_____

To-do List:
_____
_____
_____
_____
_____

A Quote:
_____
_____
_____
_____
_____

Today's Moods:

Today's Chores:
_____
_____
_____
_____

Books, Websites & Videos

Resources I can use to study today's sport:

_____
_____
_____

Start your day by watching a competition involving today's sport.

Finish the Story

Jim and Pete have decided to kayak the Everglades Wilderness Waterway. They decide to save time by trying to go down Nightmare pass. Halfway down the pass they encounter...

_____

_____

_____

_____

_____

_____

_____

Illustrate your story:

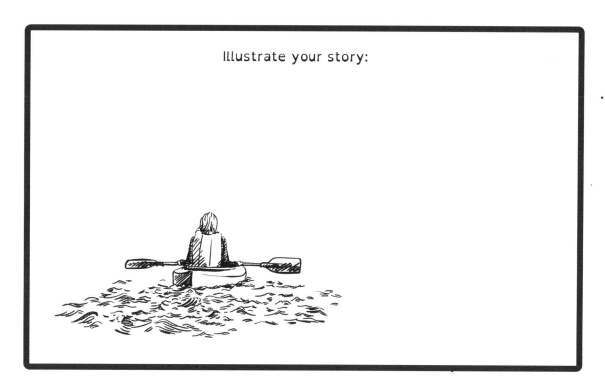

Kayaking

It's research time!

Use the Internet, books, tutorials and documentaries to study
this sport. Or go see a game or competition!

Draw any equipment needed for this sport.

Draw a player in uniform.

Draw a trophy or medal for this sport.

Where did this sport originate from?

_____

_____

How was this sport invented?

_____

_____

_____

Who are the main sponsors of the events for this sport?

_____

_____

What is the name of the largest competition where this sport is played? _____

_____

_____

_____

_____

Who is the #1 player of this sport? What makes them the best? How much money do they earn? Where do their earnings come from?

_____

_____

_____

_____

Would you like to play this sport? Why or why not?

_____

_____

What are the common injuries from playing this sport?

_____

_____

_____

Random fact about this sport.

_____

_____

_____

Say What?

Invent your own comic book font and add words to the picture

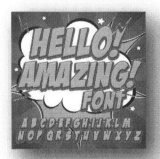 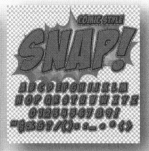 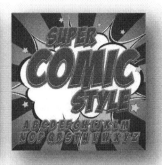 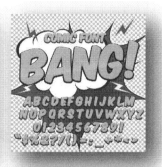

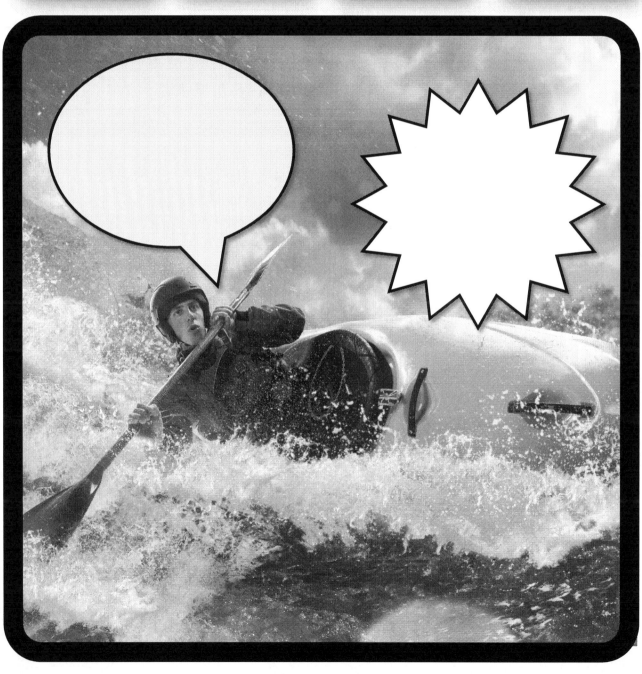

Sports News

Open a newspaper or look online!

What is happening in the world of sports today?

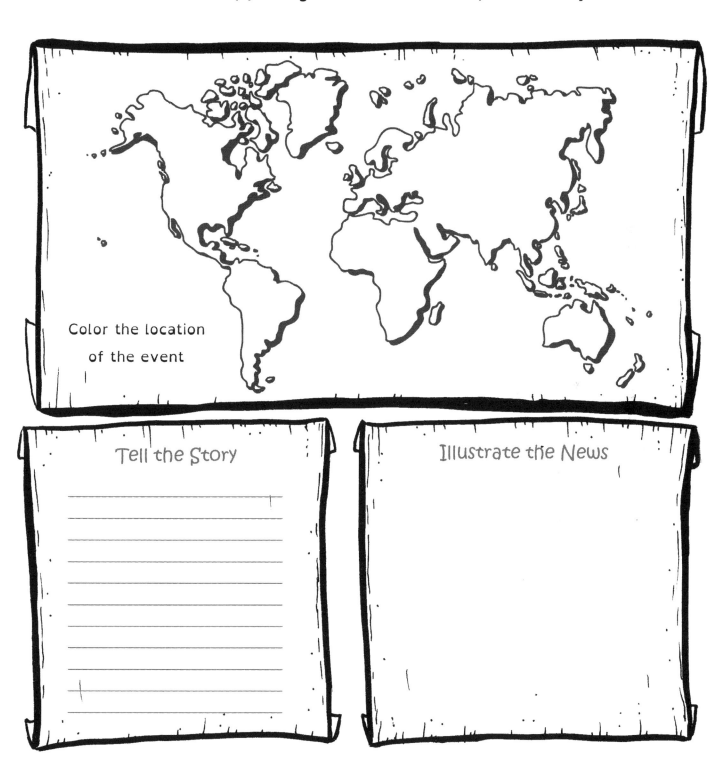

Color the location
of the event

Tell the Story

Illustrate the News

Screen Time

Watch a high-quality film, video, tutorial or sports documentary.

Title_____

Screen Time_____

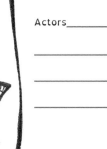

Producer_____

Actors_____

_____

_____

_____

Quotes

Draw a scene from the video.

Rating:

worst

Bad

Awful

Ok

Nice

Great

Best

Make a Comic

From the video or your imagination.

Title_____

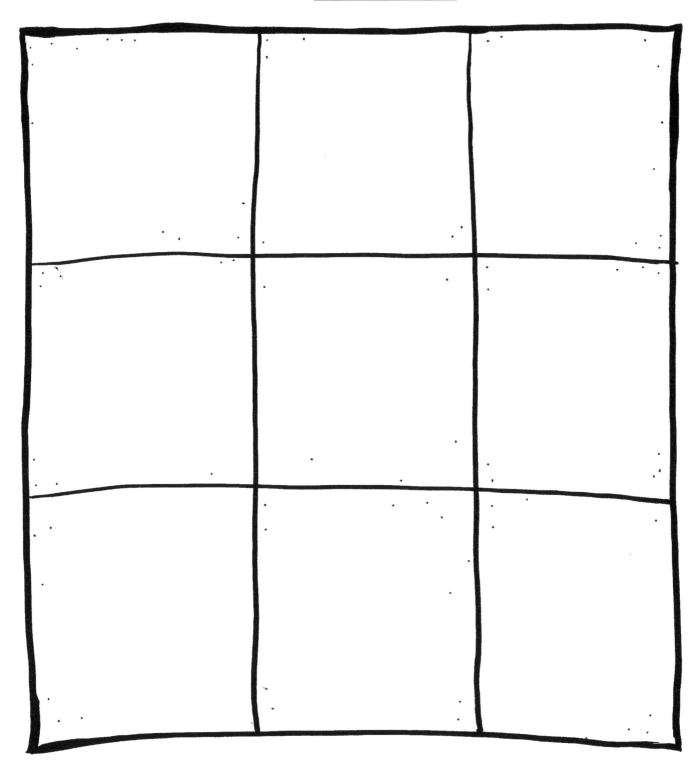

Drawing & Reading Time!

Choose a few books from your stack to focus on today.

Write down and draw anything that inspires you.

(Set a timer for 1 hour)

Free time!

Set the timer for 30 minutes and go outside to play, explore and practice a sport.

What do you plan to do on your free time?

_____

_____

What do you want to practice?

_____

_____

Do you have any goals?

_____

_____

Draw your goals!

Math Practice

Use this page for math practice,

or design a sport's field, rink or play zone

for the sport you are studying today!

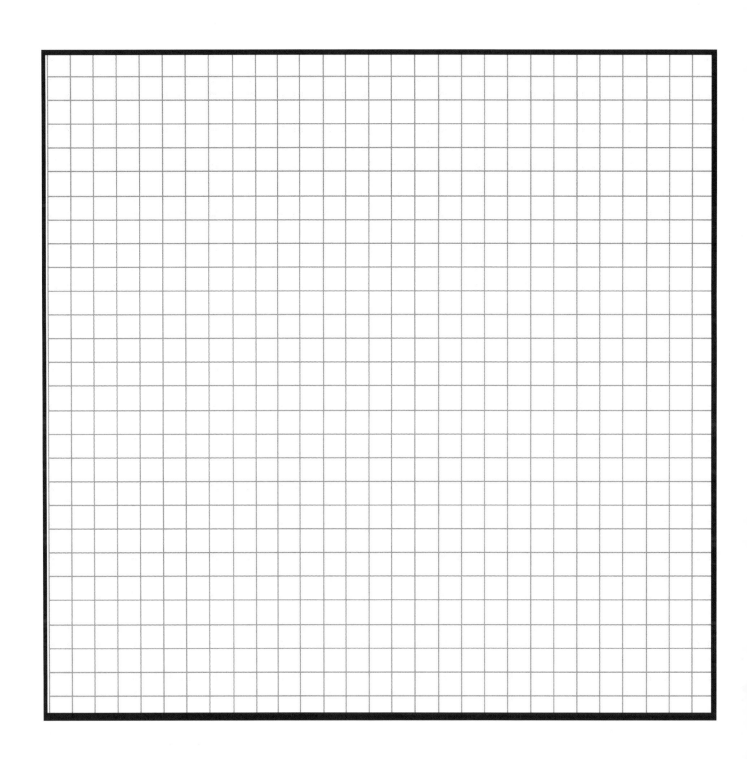

Nature Study

Take this book outside and draw anything and everything that inspires you.

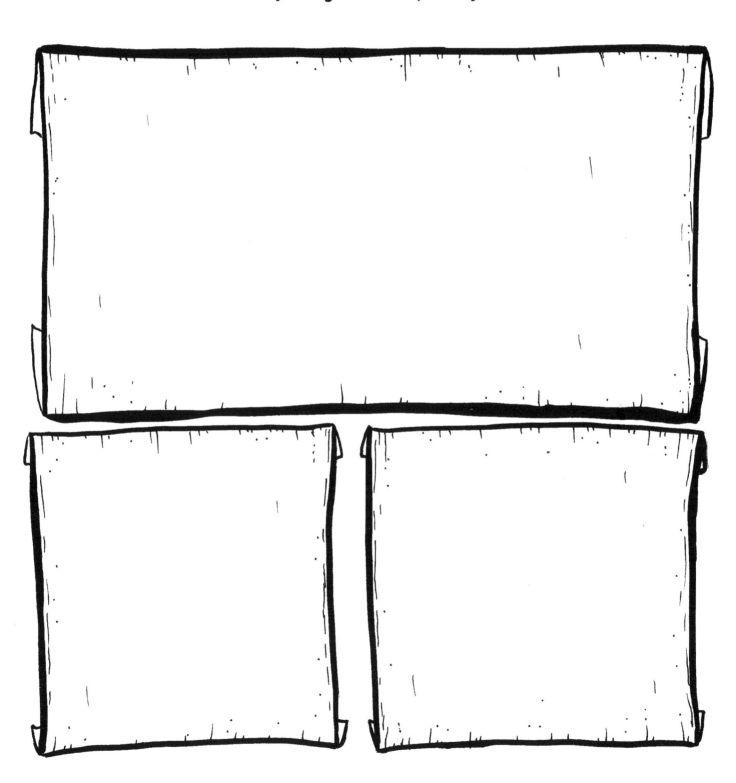

Today's Sport: Paragliding

Date:_____

To-do List:
_____
_____
_____
_____

A Quote:
_____
_____
_____
_____

Today's Moods:

Today's Chores:
_____
_____
_____
_____

Books, Websites & Videos

Resources I can use to study today's sport:

_____
_____
_____

Start your day by watching a competition involving today's sport.

Finish the Story

When Sam started paragliding 2 hours ago, the weather had been wonderful - not a cloud in sight. During the unpredictable summer weather, a storm had appeared out of nowhere. He had reached an altitude of 14,972 feet, and still had another 3,047 feet to go until he landed safely. The wind started picking up, Sam felt...

_____

_____

_____

_____

_____

_____

_____

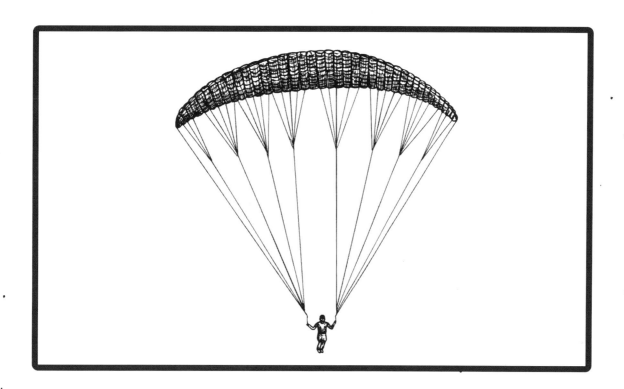

Sports Study

Paragliding

It's research time!

Use the Internet, books, tutorials and documentaries to study this sport. Or go see a game or competition!

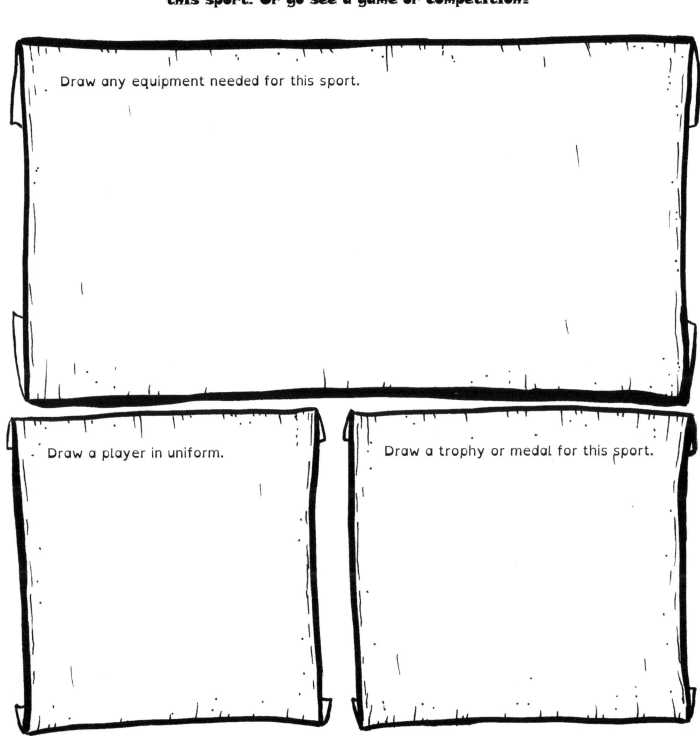

Draw any equipment needed for this sport.

Draw a player in uniform.

Draw a trophy or medal for this sport.

Where did this sport originate from?

_____

_____

How was this sport invented?

_____

_____

_____

Who are the main sponsors of the events for this sport?

_____

_____

What is the name of the largest competition where this sport is played? _____

_____

_____

_____

_____

Who is the #1 player of this sport? What makes them the best? How much money do they earn? Where do their earnings come from?

_____

_____

_____

_____

Would you like to play this sport? Why or why not?

_____

_____

What are the common injuries from playing this sport?

_____

_____

_____

Random fact about this sport.

_____

_____

_____

Say What?

Invent your own comic book font and add words to the picture

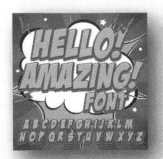
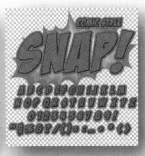
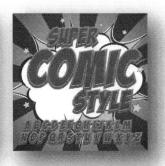
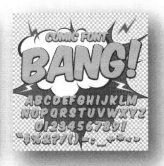

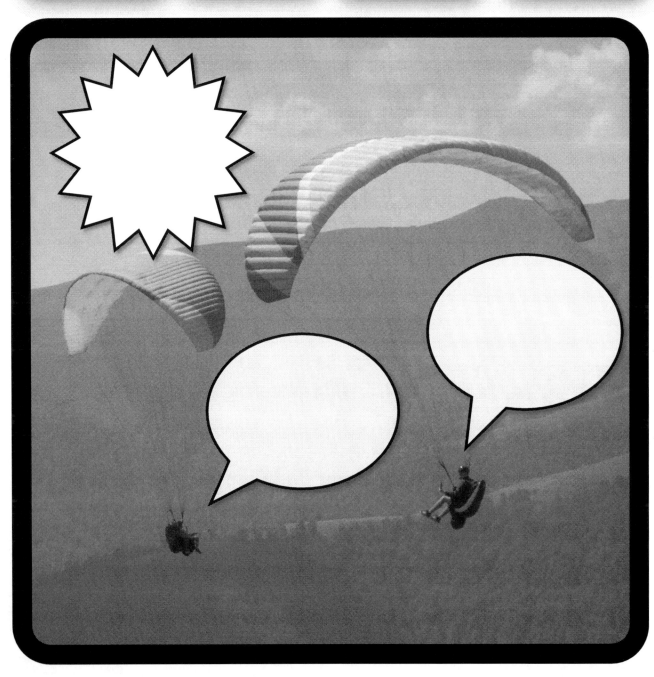

Sports News

Open a newspaper or look online!

What is happening in the world of sports today?

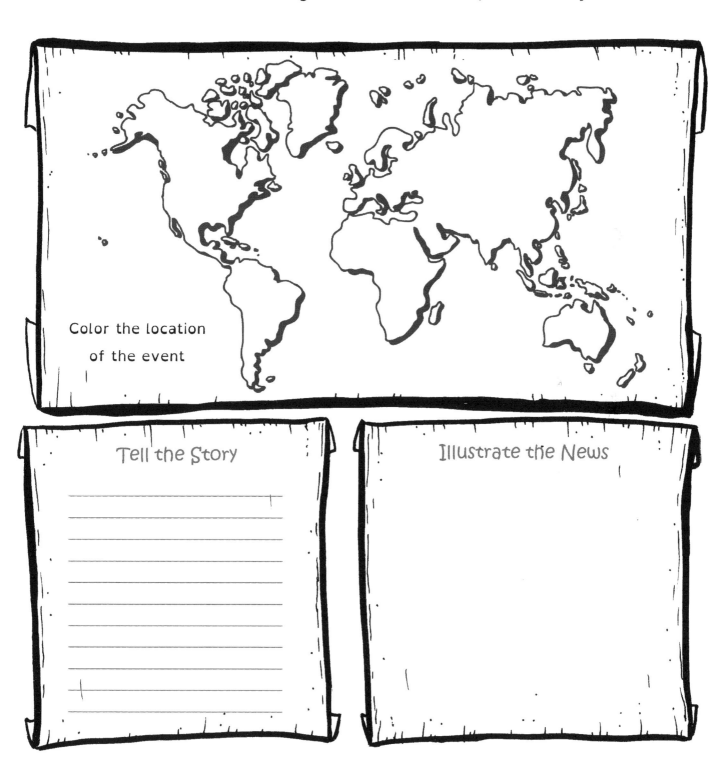

Color the location
of the event

Tell the Story

Illustrate the News

Screen Time

Watch a high-quality film, video, tutorial or sports documentary.

Title_____

Screen Time_____

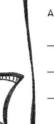

Producer_____

Actors_____

_____

_____

_____

Quotes

Draw a scene from the video.

Rating:

worst

Bad

Awful

Ok

Nice

Great

Best

Make a Comic

From the video or your imagination.

Title_____

Drawing & Reading Time!

Choose a few books from your stack to focus on today.

Write down and draw anything that inspires you.

(Set a timer for 1 hour)

Free time!

Set the timer for 30 minutes and go outside to play, explore and practice a sport.

What do you plan to do on your free time?

What do you want to practice?

Do you have any goals?

Draw your goals!

Math Practice

Use this page for math practice,

or design a sport's field, rink or play zone

for the sport you are studying today!

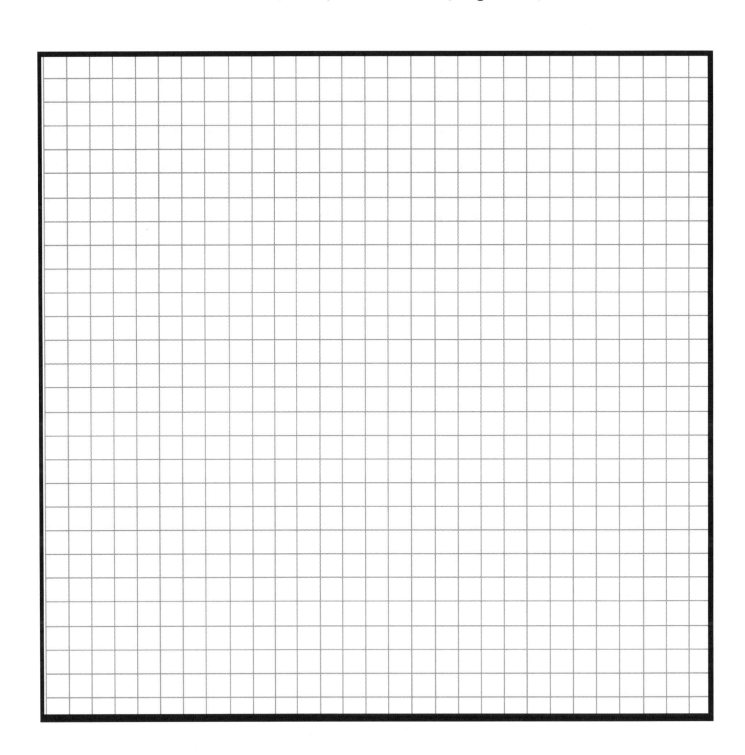

Nature Study

Take this book outside and draw anything and everything that inspires you.

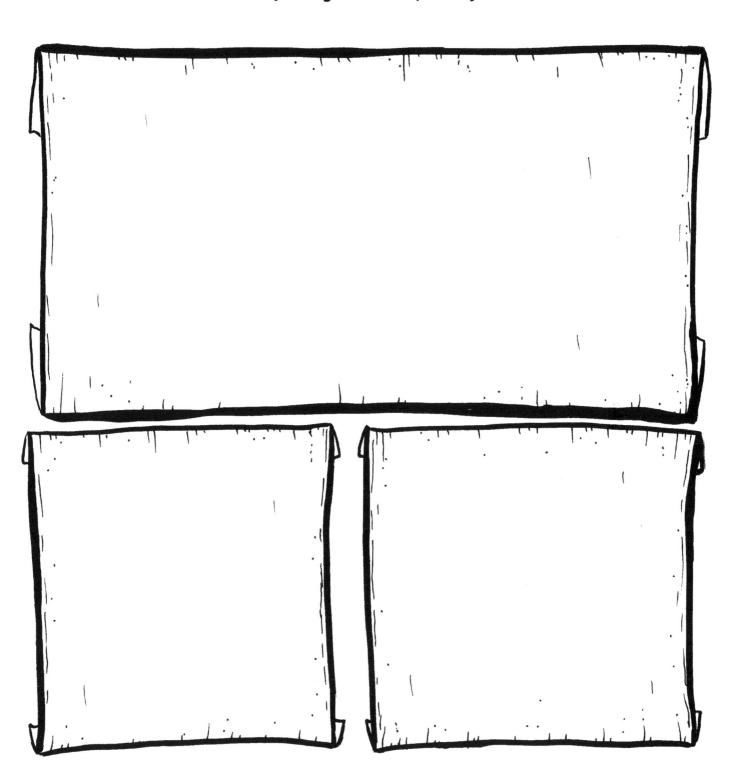

Rock Climbing

Date:_____

To-do List:

_____
_____
_____
_____

A Quote:

_____
_____
_____
_____

Today's Moods:

Today's Chores:

_____
_____
_____
_____

Books, Websites & Videos

Resources I can use to study today's sport:

_____
_____
_____

Start your day by watching a competition involving today's sport.

Finish the Story

Jasmine wants to be a solo climber and her parents are worried. You are her friend and she wants you to help her prove to her parents that it isn't so dangerous. You start to research. Do you think this is a dangerous sport? Explain to Jasmine why you feel the way you do...

_____
_____
_____
_____
_____
_____
_____

Illustrate your story:

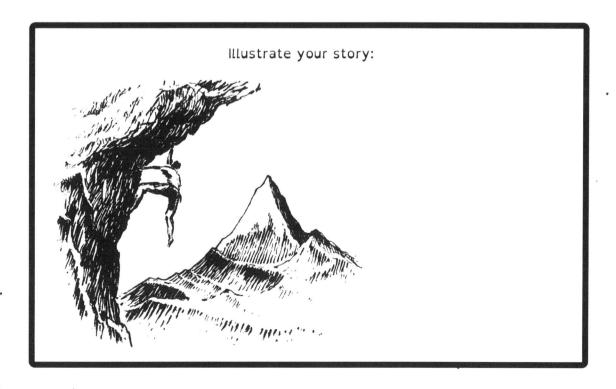

Sports Study

Rock Climbing

It's research time!

Use the Internet, books, tutorials and documentaries to study this sport. Or go see a game or competition!

Draw any equipment needed for this sport.

Draw a player in uniform.

Draw a trophy or medal for this sport.

Where did this sport originate from?

_____

_____

How was this sport invented?

_____

_____

_____

Who are the main sponsors of the events for this sport?

_____

_____

What is the name of the largest competition where this sport is played? _____

_____

_____

_____

_____

Who is the #1 player of this sport? What makes them the best? How much money do they earn? Where do their earnings come from?

_____

_____

_____

_____

Would you like to play this sport? Why or why not?

_____

_____

What are the common injuries from playing this sport?

_____

_____

_____

_____

Random fact about this sport.

_____

_____

_____

Say What?

Invent your own comic book font and add words to the picture

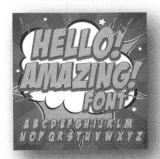
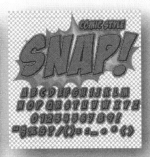
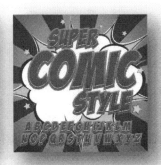
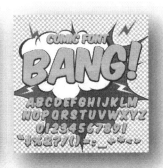

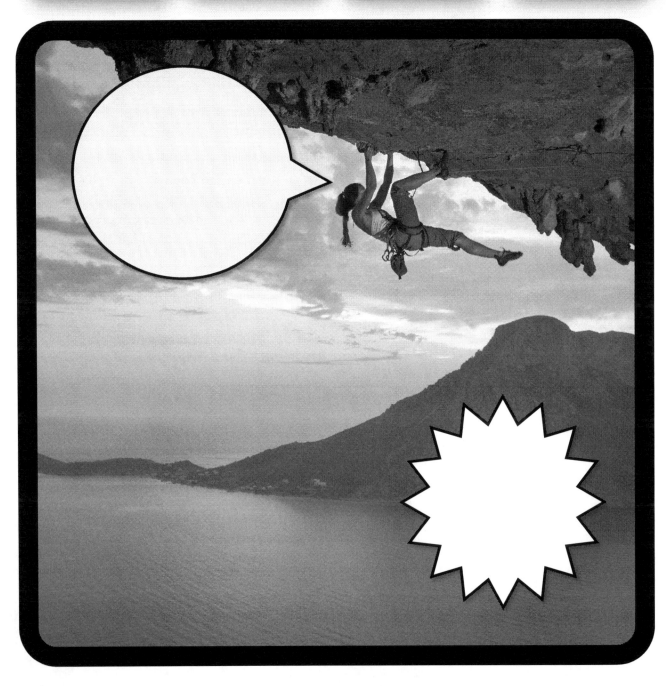

Sports News

Open a newspaper or look online!

What is happening in the world of sports today?

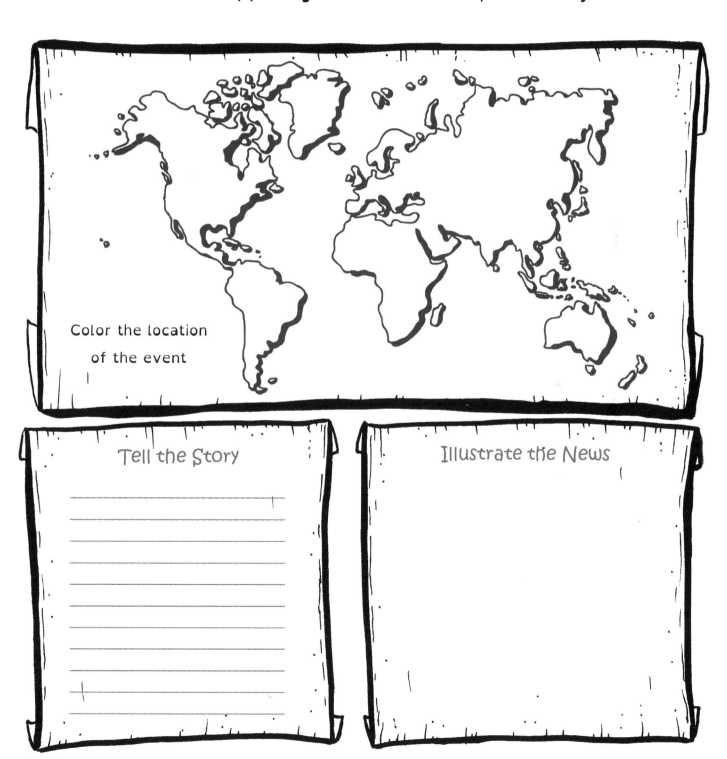

Color the location
of the event

Tell the Story

Illustrate the News

Screen Time

Watch a high-quality film, video, tutorial or sports documentary.

Title_____

Screen Time_____

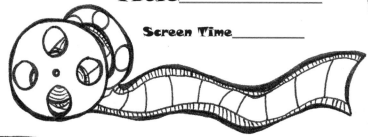

Producer_____

Actors_____

_____

_____

_____

Quotes

Draw a scene from the video.

Rating:

worst

Bad

Awful

Ok

Nice

Great

Best

Make a Comic

From the video or your imagination.

Title_____

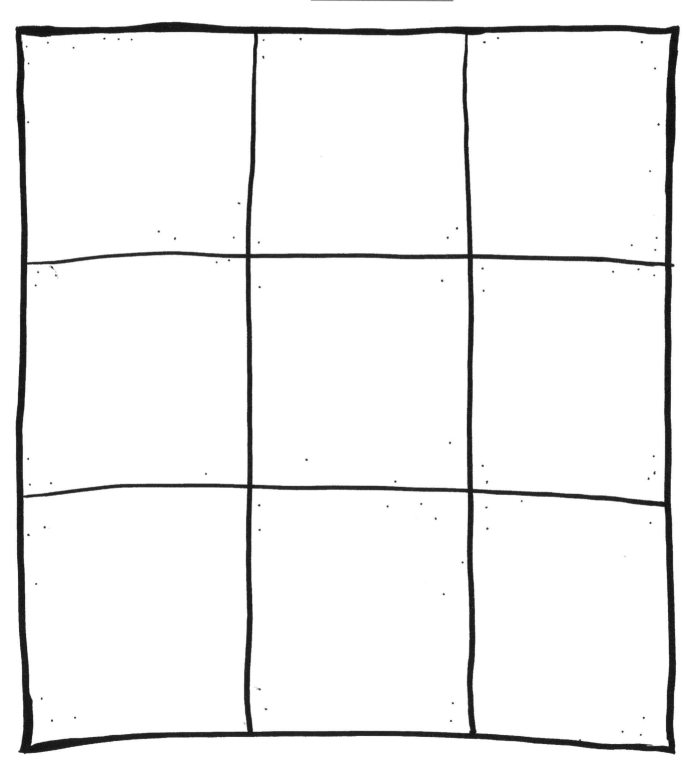

Drawing & Reading Time!

Choose a few books from your stack to focus on today.

Write down and draw anything that inspires you.

(Set a timer for 1 hour)

Free time!

Set the timer for 30 minutes and go outside to play, explore and practice a sport.

What do you plan to do on your free time?

What do you want to practice?

Do you have any goals?

Draw your goals!

Math Practice

Use this page for math practice,

or design a sport's field, rink or play zone

for the sport you are studying today!

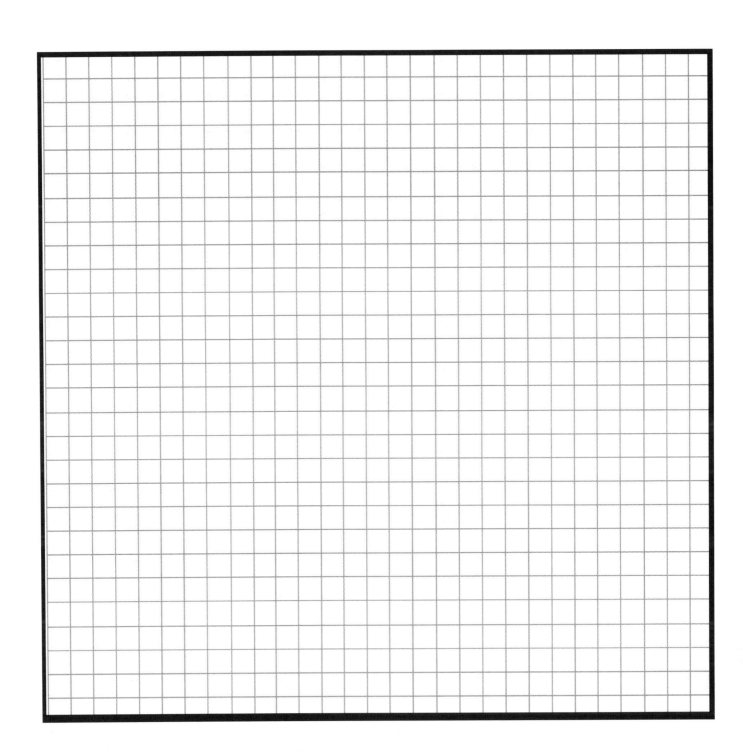

Nature Study

Take this book outside and draw anything and everything that inspires you.

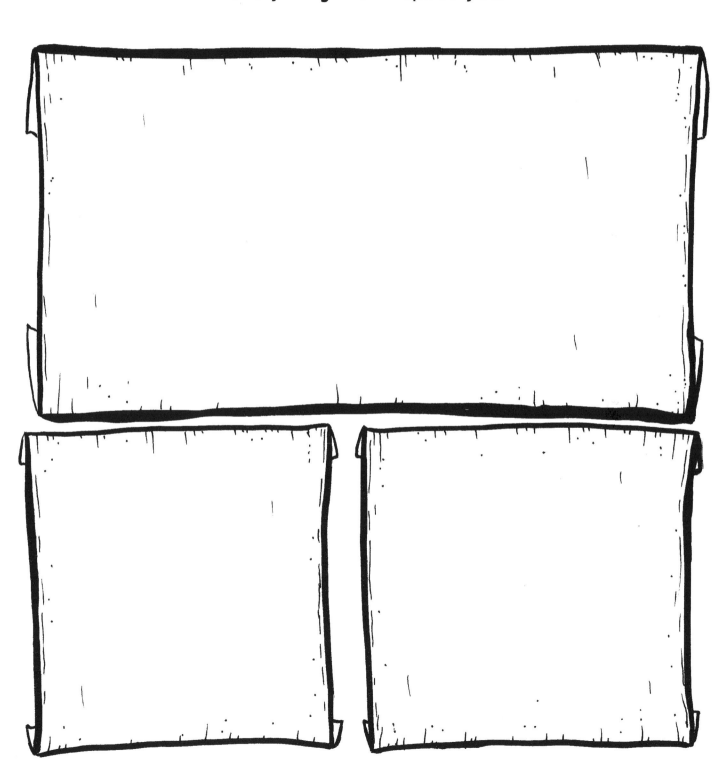

Today's Sport: Snowboarding

Date:_____

To-do List:
_____
_____
_____
_____
_____

A Quote:
_____
_____
_____
_____
_____

Today's Moods:

Today's Chores:
_____
_____
_____
_____

Books, Websites & Videos

Resources I can use to study today's sport:

_____
_____
_____

Start your day by watching a competition involving today's sport.

Math & Research Challenge

In order to be one of the twelve competitors moving on to the final round, Shaun has to score at least a 97.8 by performing various tricks on the halfpipe. Besides a double cork, what are some other tricks Shaun can perform to help his score?

Solve the challenge:

_____

_____

_____

_____

_____

_____

ANSWER:

_____

Illustrate your answer:

Sports Study

Snowboarding

It's research time!

Use the Internet, books, tutorials and documentaries to study this sport. Or go see a game or competition!

Draw any equipment needed for this sport.

Draw a player in uniform.

Draw a trophy or medal for this sport.

Where did this sport originate from?

_____

_____

How was this sport invented?

_____

_____

_____

Who are the main sponsors of the events for this sport?

_____

_____

What is the name of the largest competition where this sport is played? _____

_____

_____

_____

_____

Who is the #1 player of this sport? What makes them the best? How much money do they earn? Where do their earnings come from?

_____

_____

_____

_____

Would you like to play this sport? Why or why not?

_____

_____

What are the common injuries from playing this sport?

_____

_____

_____

Random fact about this sport.

_____

_____

_____

Say What?

Invent your own comic book font and add words to the picture

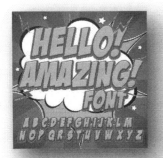
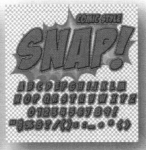
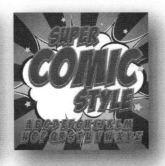
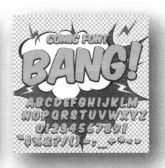

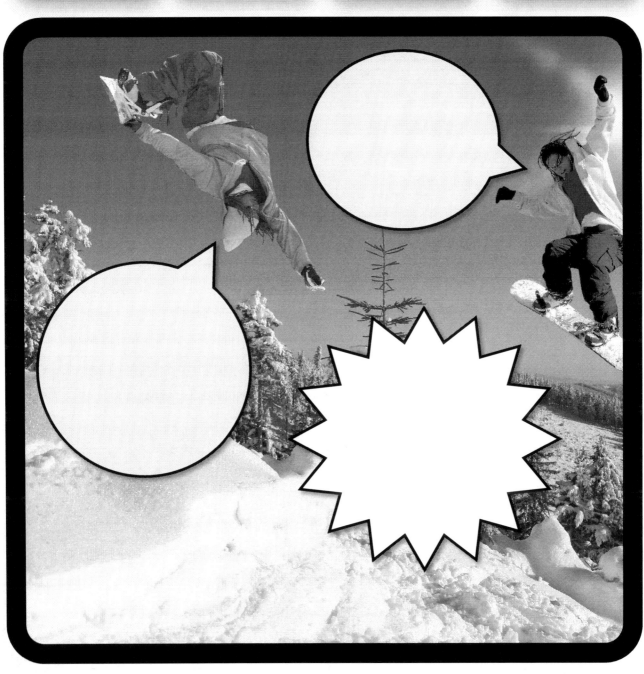

Sports News

Open a newspaper or look online!

What is happening in the world of sports today?

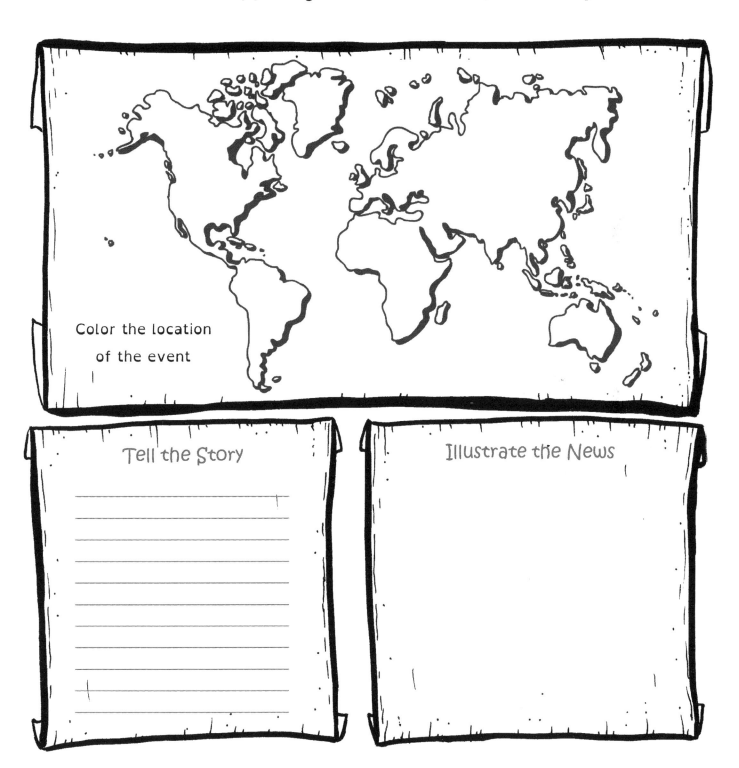

Color the location
of the event

Tell the Story

Illustrate the News

Screen Time

Watch a high-quality film, video, tutorial or sports documentary.

Title_____

Screen Time_____

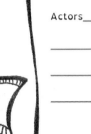

Producer_____

Actors_____

_____

_____

_____

Quotes

Draw a scene from the video.

Rating:

worst

Bad

Awful

Ok

Nice

Great

Best

Make a Comic

From the video or your imagination.

Title_____

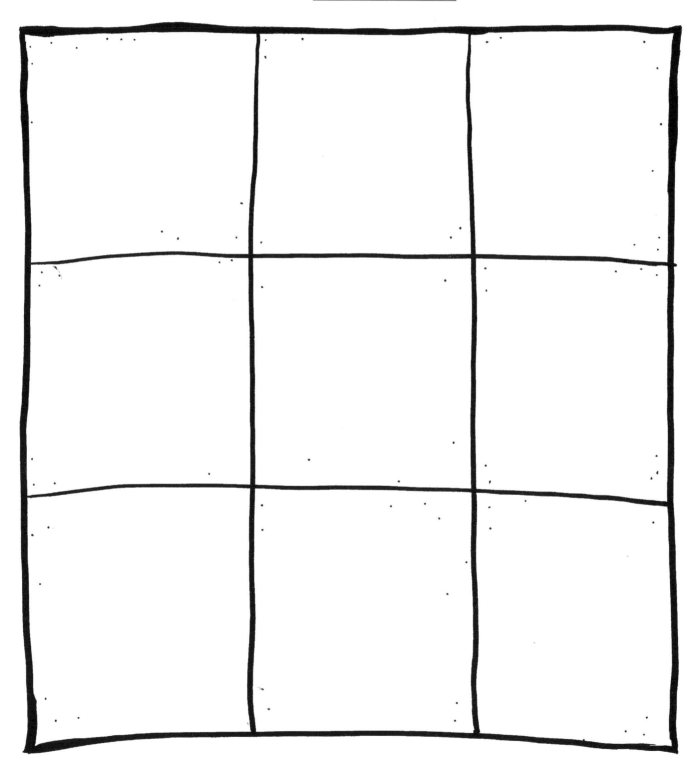

Drawing & Reading Time!

Choose a few books from your stack to focus on today.

Write down and draw anything that inspires you.

(Set a timer for 1 hour)

Free time!

Set the timer for 30 minutes and go outside to play, explore and practice a sport.

What do you plan to do on your free time?

What do you want to practice?

Do you have any goals?

Draw your goals!

Math Practice

Use this page for math practice,
or design a sport's field, rink or play zone
for the sport you are studying today!

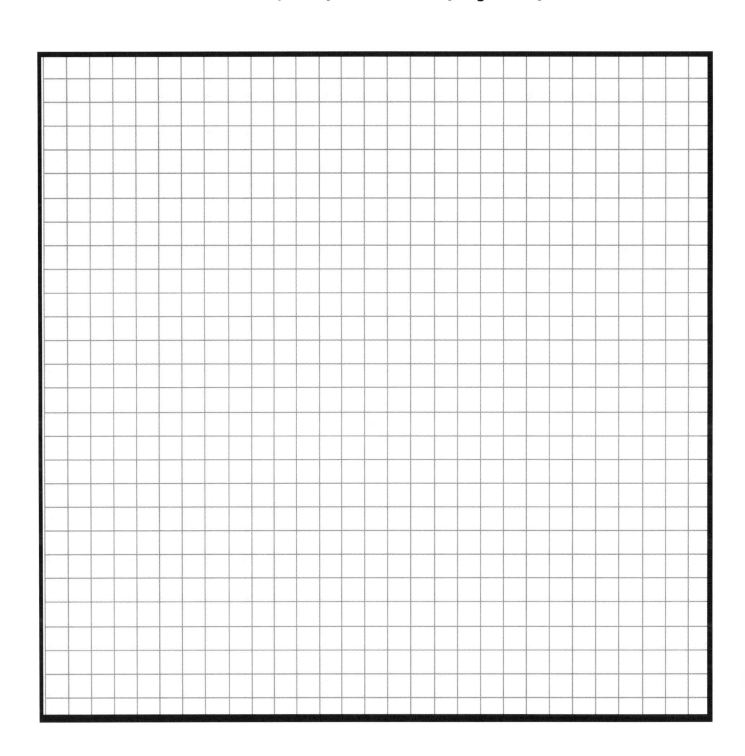

Nature Study

Take this book outside and draw anything and
everything that inspires you.

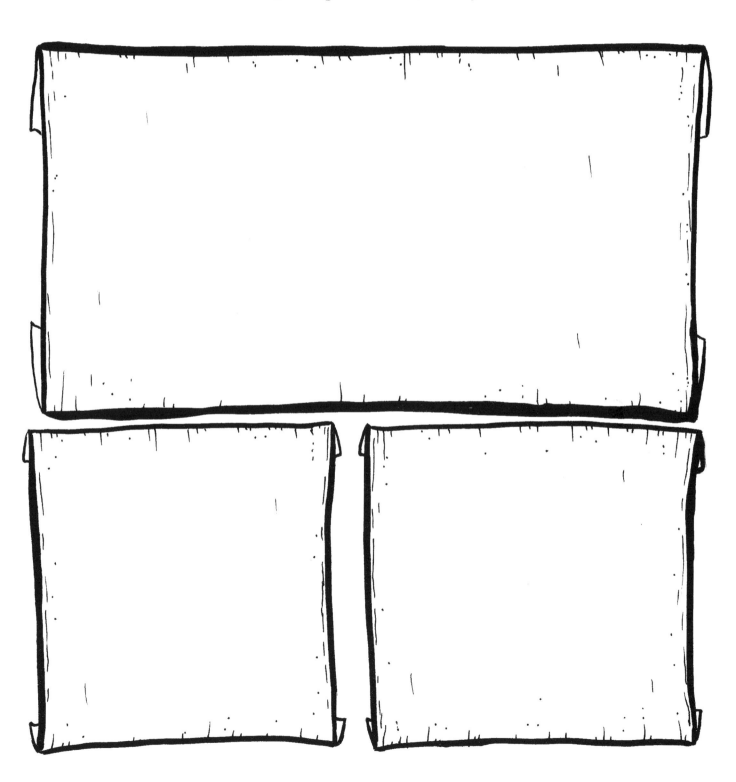

Today's Sport: Swimming

Date:_____

To-do List:

_____
_____
_____
_____
_____

A Quote:

_____
_____
_____
_____

Today's Moods:

Today's Chores:

_____
_____
_____
_____

Books, Websites & Videos

Resources I can use to study today's sport:

_____
_____
_____

Start your day by watching a competition involving today's sport.

Math & Research Challenge

John was working to improve his swimming scores at each meet. His last three meets have averaged 31.2 seconds for every 25 meters. So far this meet, he has scored a 29.7 and a 30.2. What does he need on his last three races to beat his meet average?

Solve the challenge:

_____

_____

_____

_____

_____

_____

ANSWER:

_____

Illustrate your answer:

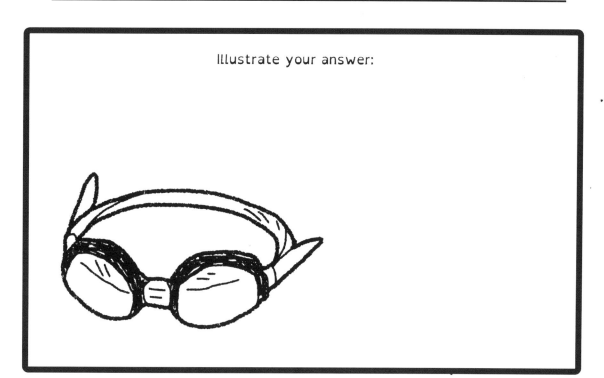

Sports Study

Swimming

It's research time!

Use the Internet, books, tutorials and documentaries to study this sport. Or go see a game or competition!

Draw any equipment needed for this sport.

Draw a player in uniform.

Draw a trophy or medal for this sport.

Where did this sport originate from?

_____

_____

How was this sport invented?

_____

_____

_____

Who are the main sponsors of the events for this sport?

_____

_____

What is the name of the largest competition where this sport is played? _____

_____

_____

_____

_____

Who is the #1 player of this sport? What makes them the best? How much money do they earn? Where do their earnings come from?

_____

_____

_____

_____

Would you like to play this sport? Why or why not?

_____

_____

What are the common injuries from playing this sport?

_____

_____

_____

_____

Random fact about this sport.

_____

_____

_____

Say What?

Invent your own comic book font and add words to the picture

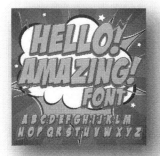
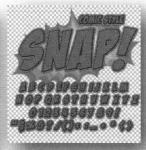
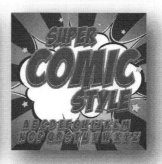
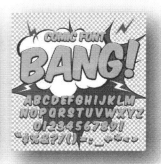

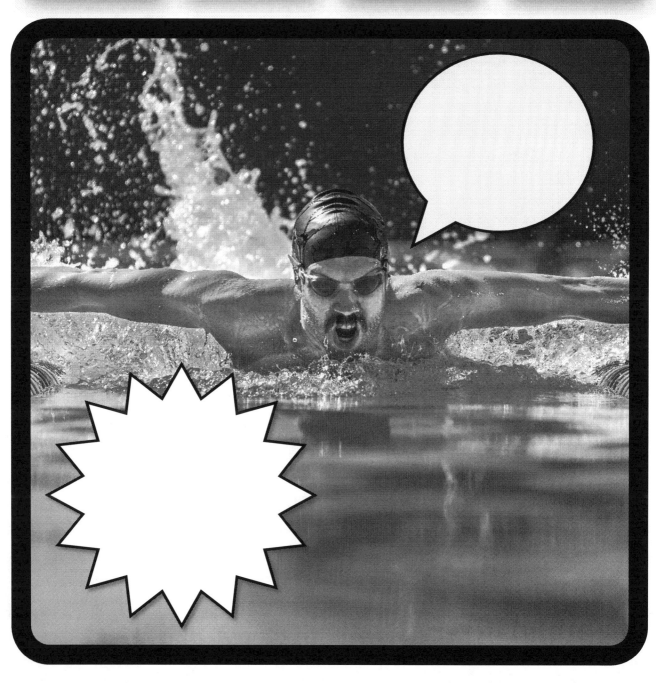

Sports News

Open a newspaper or look online!

What is happening in the world of sports today?

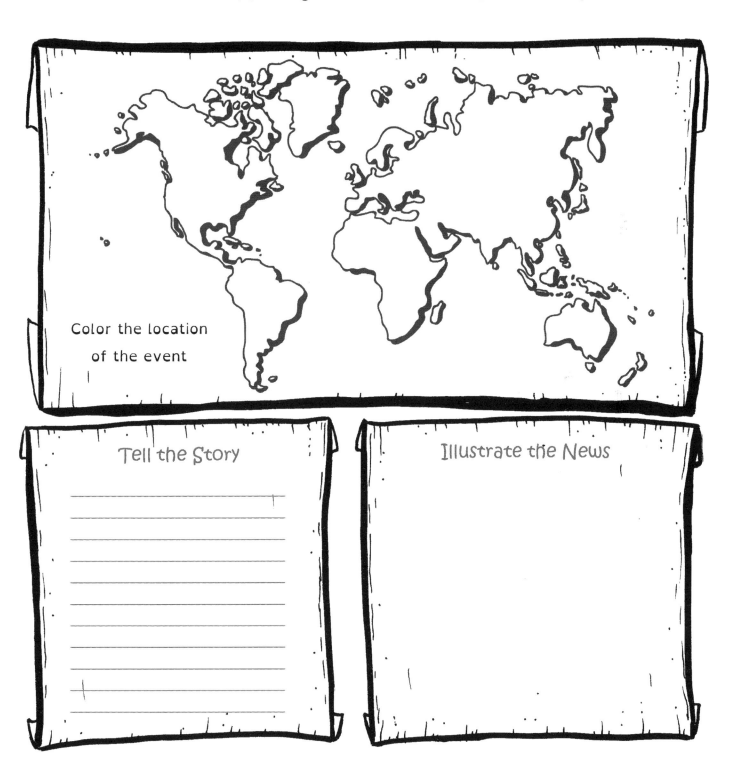

Color the location
of the event

Tell the Story

Illustrate the News

Screen Time

Watch a high-quality film, video, tutorial or sports documentary.

Title_____

Screen Time_____

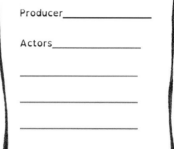

Producer_____

Actors_____

_____

_____

_____

_____

Quotes

Draw a scene from the video.

Rating:

worst

Bad

Awful

Ok

Nice

Great

Best

Make a Comic

From the video or your imagination.

Title_____

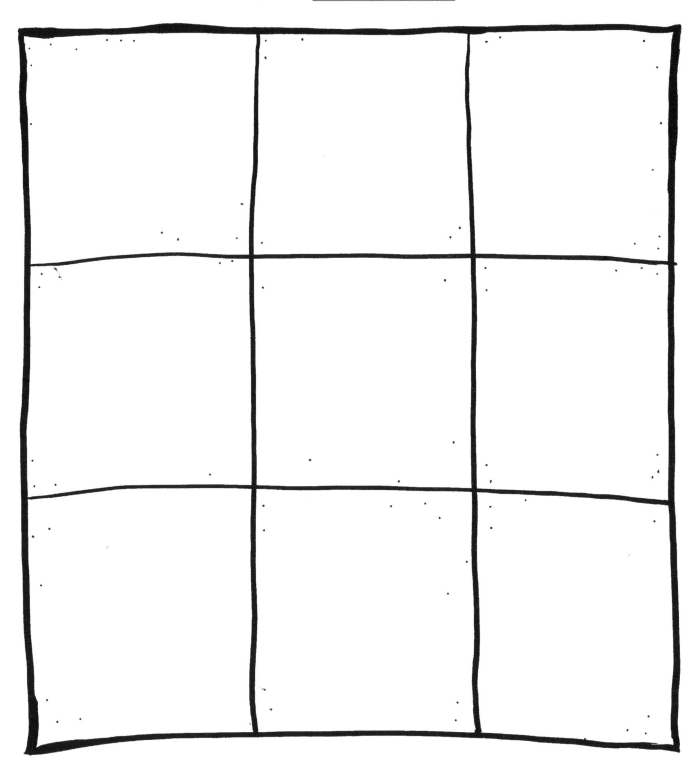

Drawing & Reading Time!

Choose a few books from your stack to focus on today.

Write down and draw anything that inspires you.

(Set a timer for 1 hour)

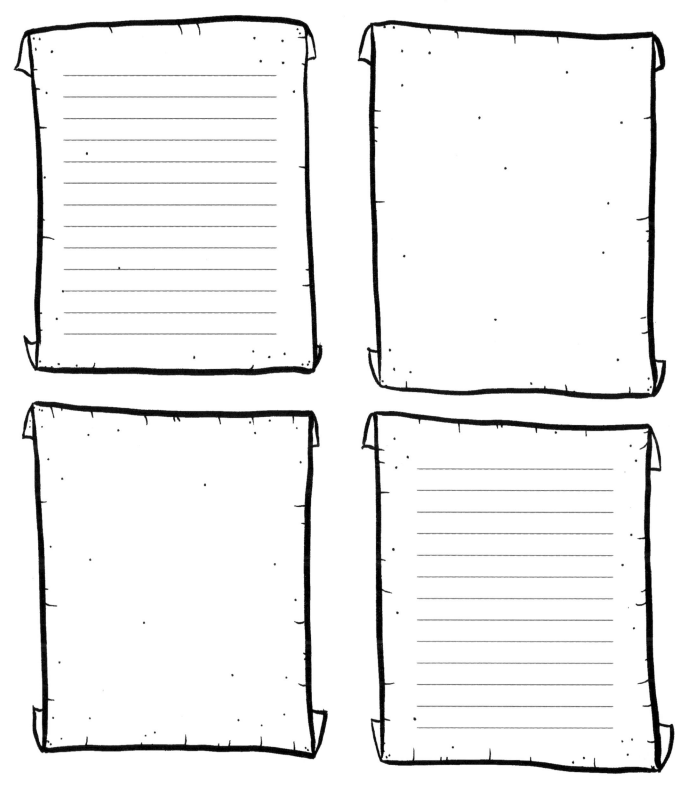

Free time!

Set the timer for 30 minutes and go outside to play, explore and practice a sport.

What do you plan to do on your free time?

_____

_____

What do you want to practice?

_____

_____

Do you have any goals?

_____

_____

Draw your goals!

Math Practice

Use this page for math practice,

or design a sport's field, rink or play zone

for the sport you are studying today!

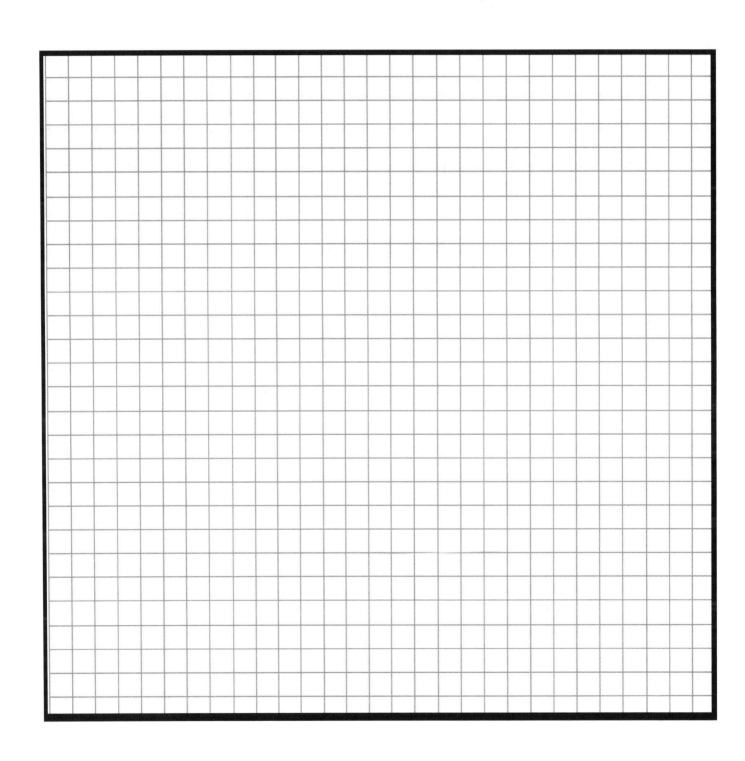

Nature Study

Take this book outside and draw anything and
everything that inspires you.

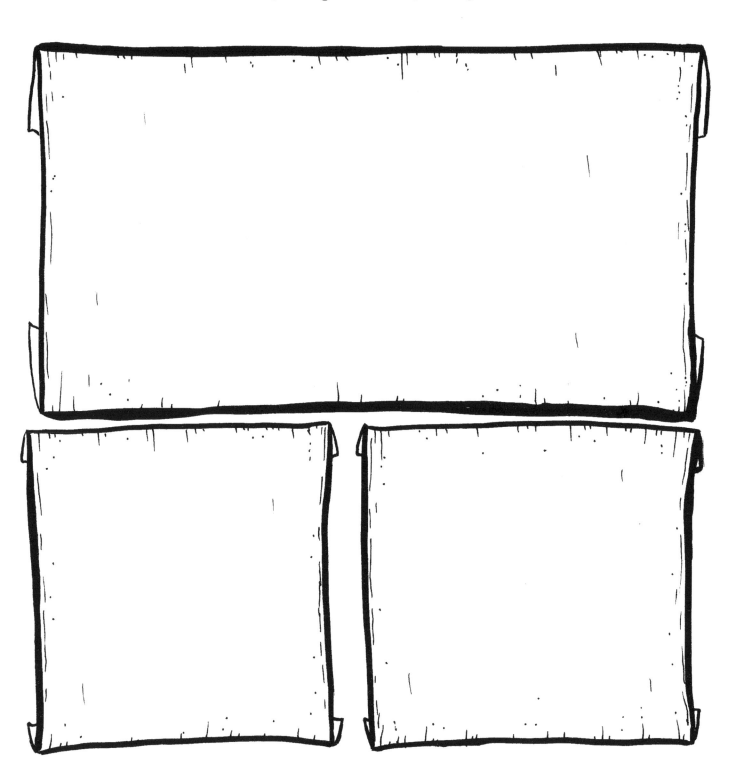

Today's Sport: Soccer

Date:_____

To-do List:
_____
_____
_____
_____

A Quote:
_____
_____
_____
_____

Today's Moods:

Today's Chores:
_____
_____
_____
_____

Books, Websites & Videos

Resources I can use to study today's sport:

_____
_____
_____

Start your day by watching a competition involving today's sport.

Finish the Story

Luke ran down the left side of the soccer field, stepping around a defender to receive a pass from his teammate, Jake. He lunged forward, just catching the soccer ball with the tip of his left foot. As he took control of the ball, he sped past the last defender toward the goal...

_____

_____

_____

_____

_____

_____

_____

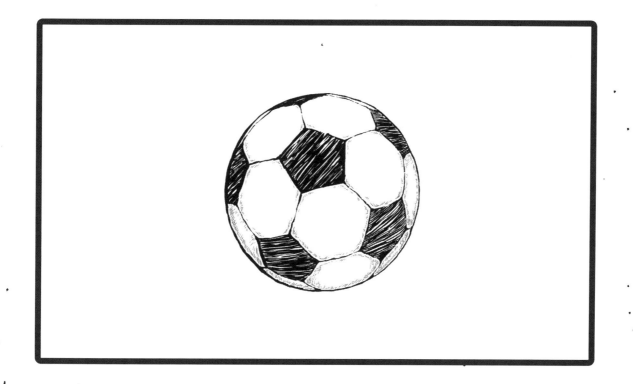

Sports Study

Soccer

It's research time!

Use the Internet, books, tutorials and documentaries to study this sport. Or go see a game or competition!

Draw any equipment needed for this sport.

Draw a player in uniform.

Draw a trophy or medal for this sport.

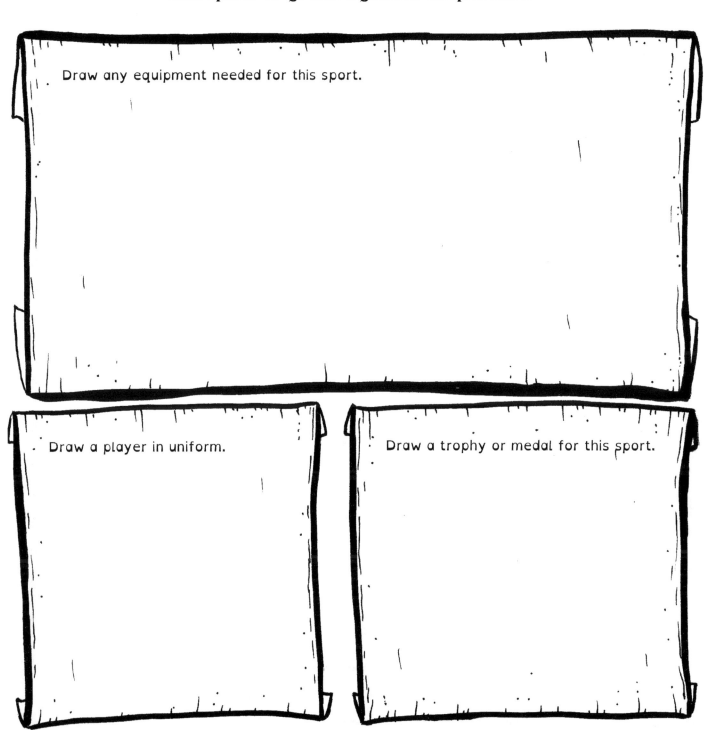

Where did this sport originate from?

_____

_____

How was this sport invented?

_____

_____

_____

Who are the main sponsors of the events for this sport?

_____

_____

What is the name of the largest competition where this sport is played? _____

_____

_____

_____

_____

Who is the #1 player of this sport? What makes them the best? How much money do they earn? Where do their earnings come from?

_____

_____

_____

_____

Would you like to play this sport? Why or why not?

_____

_____

What are the common injuries from playing this sport?

_____

_____

_____

Random fact about this sport.

_____

_____

_____

Say What?

Invent your own comic book font and add words to the picture

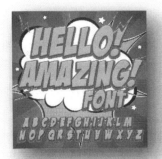
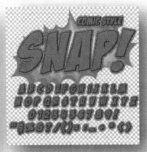
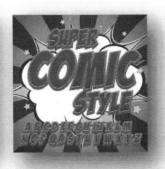
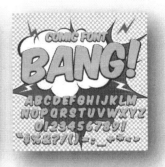

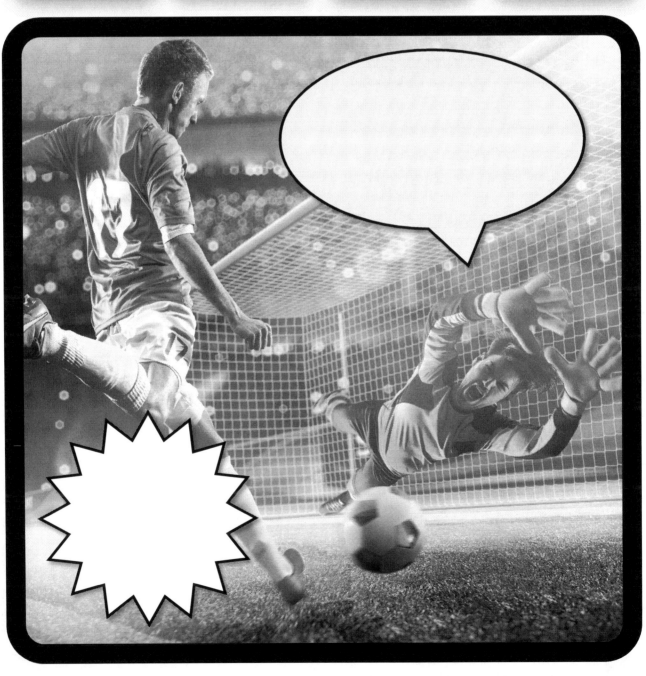

Sports News

Open a newspaper or look online!

What is happening in the world of sports today?

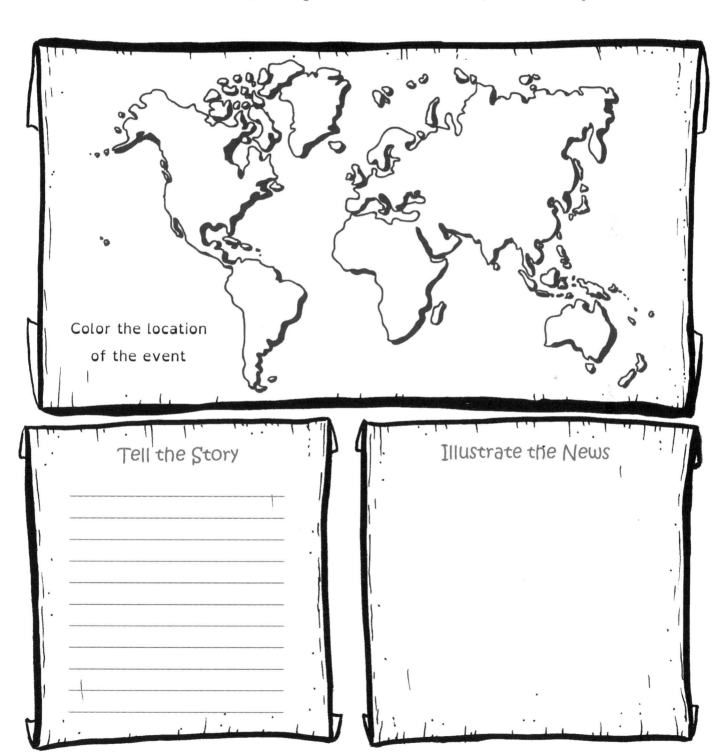

Color the location
of the event

Tell the Story

Illustrate the News

Screen Time

Watch a high-quality film, video, tutorial or sports documentary.

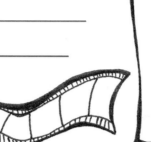

Title_____

Screen Time_____

Producer_____

Actors_____

_____

_____

_____

Quotes

Draw a scene from the video.

Rating:

worst

Bad

Awful

Ok

Nice

Great

Best

Make a Comic

From the video or your imagination.

Title_____

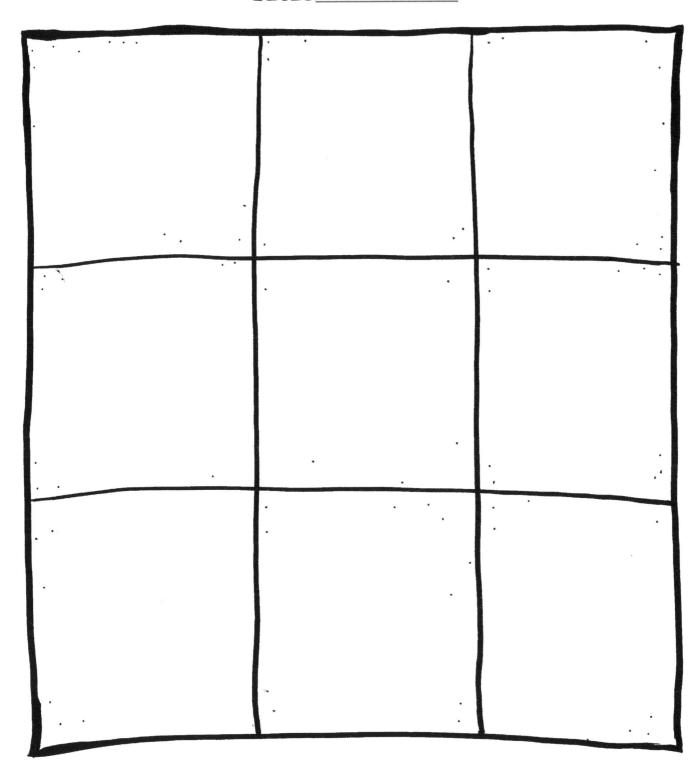

Drawing & Reading Time!

Choose a few books from your stack to focus on today.

Write down and draw anything that inspires you.

(Set a timer for 1 hour)

Free time!

Set the timer for 30 minutes and go outside to play, explore and practice a sport.

What do you plan to do on your free time?

_____

_____

What do you want to practice?

_____

_____

Do you have any goals?

_____

_____

Draw your goals!

Math Practice

Use this page for math practice,

or design a sport's field, rink or play zone

for the sport you are studying today!

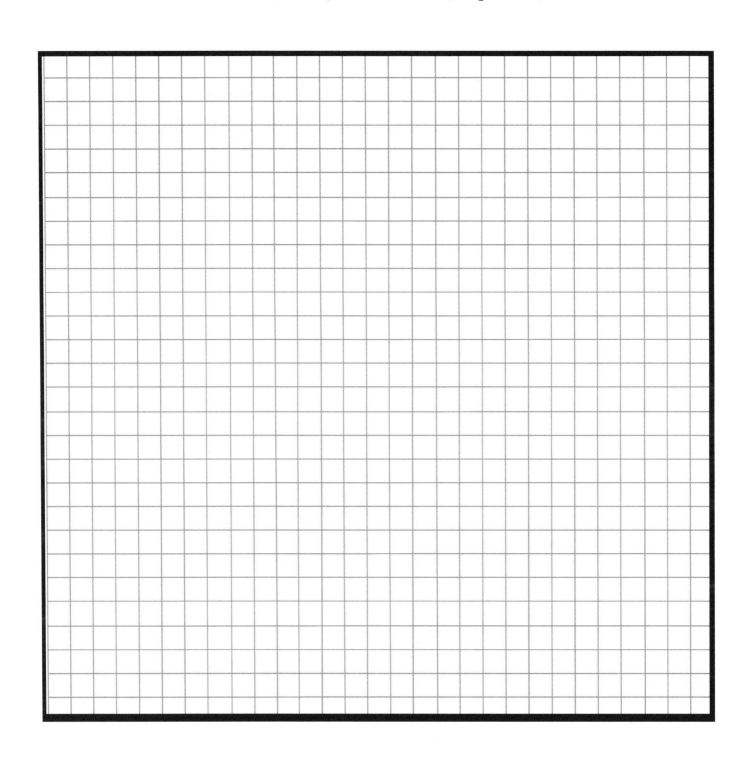

Nature Study

Take this book outside and draw anything and everything that inspires you.

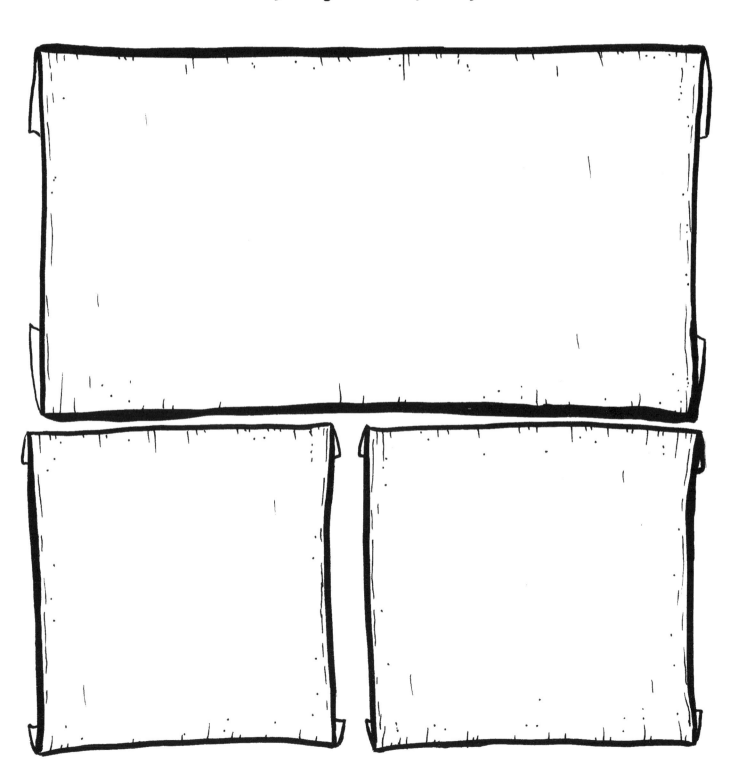

Today's Sport: Scuba Diving

Date:_____

To-do List:
_____
_____
_____
_____
_____

A Quote:
_____
_____
_____
_____

Today's Moods:

Today's Chores:
_____
_____
_____
_____

Books, Websites & Videos

Resources I can use to study today's sport:

_____
_____
_____

Start your day by watching a competition involving today's sport.

Math & Research Challenge

30 meters down, a scuba diver uses air four times faster than on the surface. If a diver has an oxygen tank that should last for 2.5 hours on the surface, how long will it last the diver at 30 meters below the surface?

Solve the challenge:

_____
_____
_____
_____
_____
_____

ANSWER:

_____

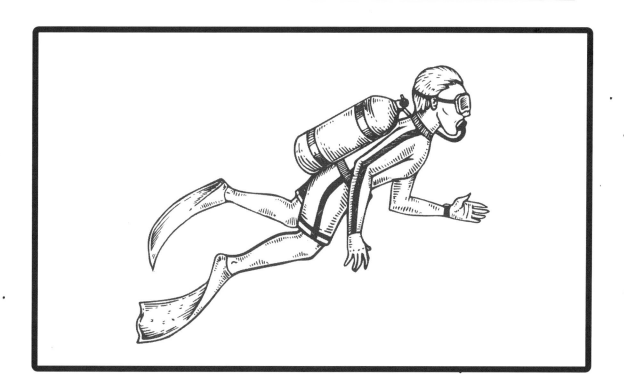

Sports Study

Scuba Diving

It's research time!

Use the Internet, books, tutorials and documentaries to study this sport. Or go see a game or competition!

Draw any equipment needed for this sport.

Draw a player in uniform.

Draw a trophy or medal for this sport.

Where did this sport originate from?

_____

_____

How was this sport invented?

_____

_____

_____

Who are the main sponsors of the events for this sport?

_____

_____

What is the name of the largest competition where this sport is played? _____

_____

_____

_____

_____

Who is the #1 player of this sport? What makes them the best? How much money do they earn? Where do their earnings come from?

_____

_____

_____

_____

Would you like to play this sport? Why or why not?

_____

_____

What are the common injuries from playing this sport?

_____

_____

_____

Random fact about this sport.

_____

_____

_____

Say What?

Invent your own comic book font and add words to the picture

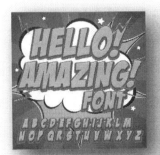
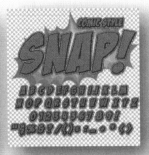
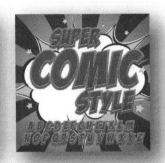
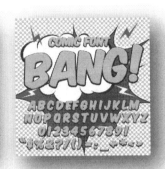

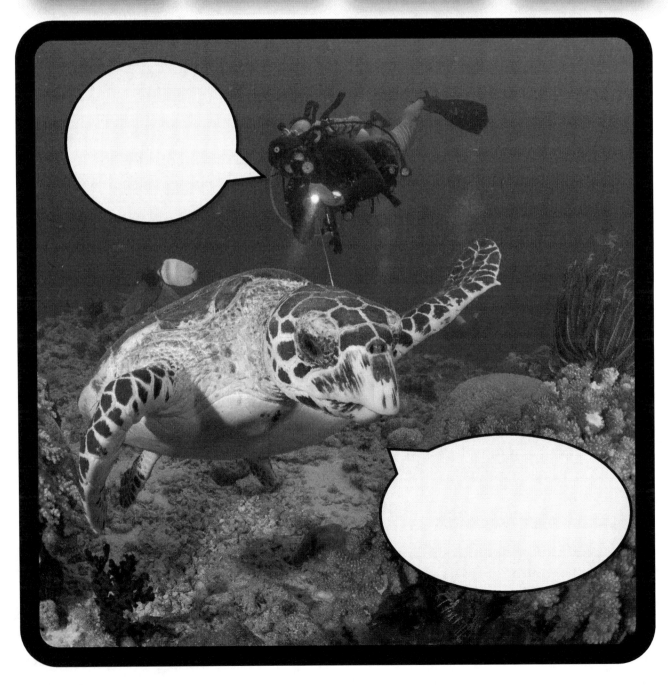

Sports News

Open a newspaper or look online!

What is happening in the world of sports today?

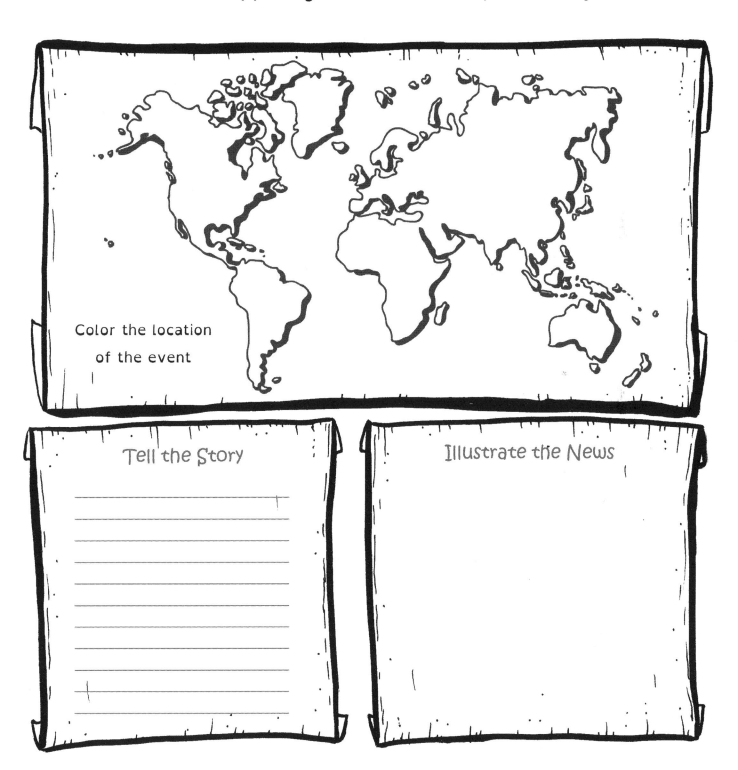

Color the location
of the event

Tell the Story

Illustrate the News

Screen Time

Watch a high-quality film, video, tutorial or sports documentary.

Title_____

Screen Time_____

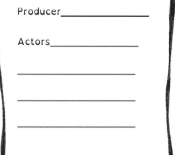

Producer_____

Actors_____

_____

_____

_____

Quotes

Draw a scene from the video.

Rating:

worst

Bad

Awful

Ok

Nice

Great

Best

Make a Comic

From the video or your imagination.

Title_____

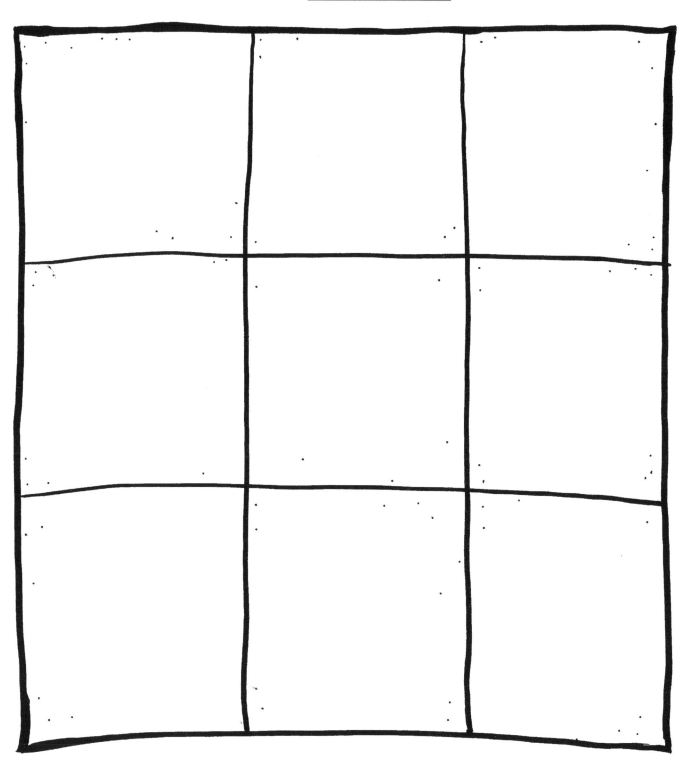

Drawing & Reading Time!

Choose a few books from your stack to focus on today.

Write down and draw anything that inspires you.

(Set a timer for 1 hour)

Free time!

Set the timer for 30 minutes and go outside to play, explore and practice a sport.

What do you plan to do on your free time?

_____

_____

What do you want to practice?

_____

_____

Do you have any goals?

_____

_____

Draw your goals!

Math Practice

Use this page for math practice,

or design a sport's field, rink or play zone

for the sport you are studying today!

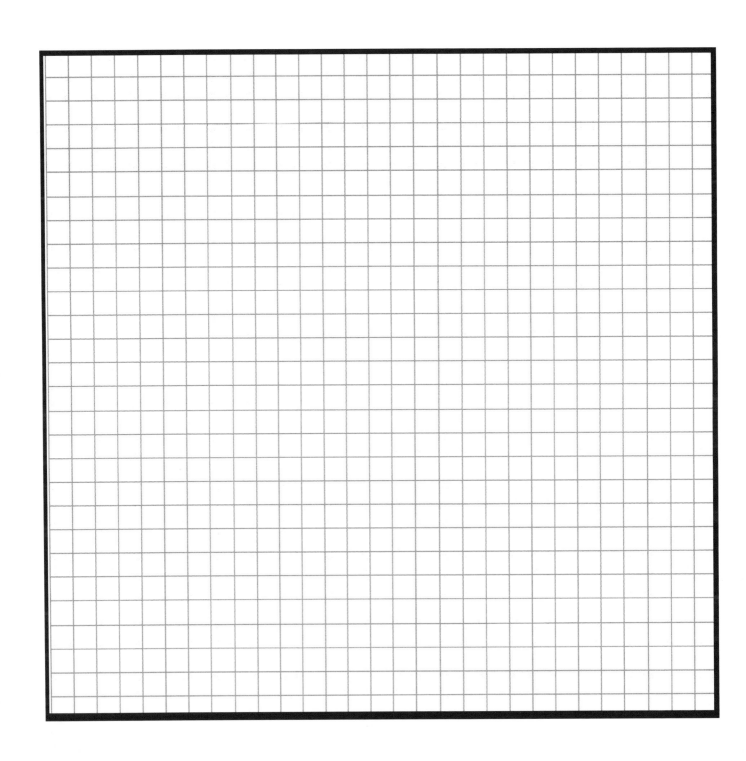

Nature Study

Take this book outside and draw anything and everything that inspires you.

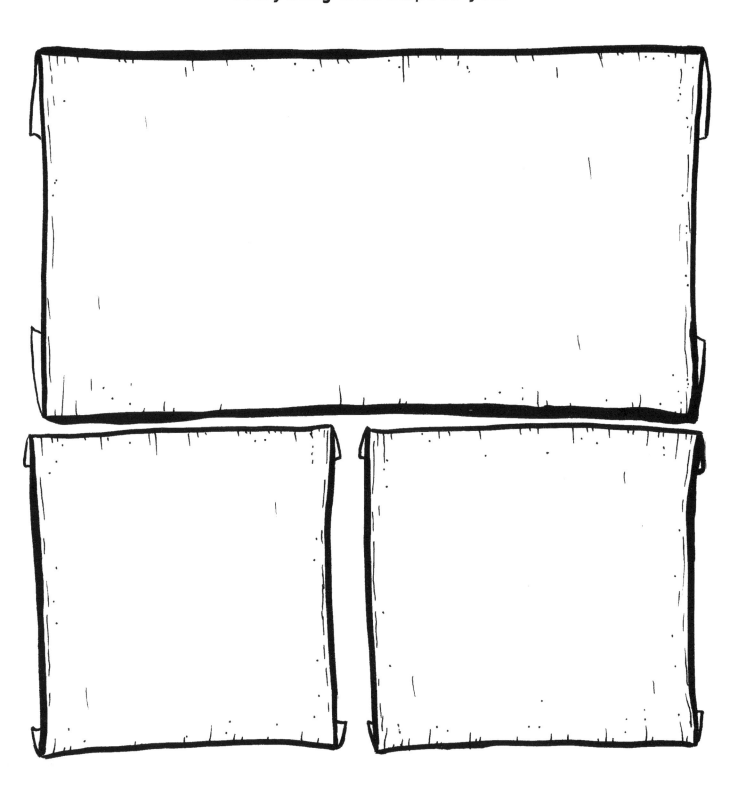

Today's Sport: _____

Date:_____

To-do List:
_____
_____
_____
_____
_____

A Quote:
_____
_____
_____
_____

Today's Moods:

Today's Chores:
_____
_____
_____
_____

Books, Websites & Videos

Resources I can use to study today's sport:

_____
_____
_____

Start your day by watching a competition involving today's sport.

Finish the Story

I'm almost finished with my Athlete's Fun-Schooling Journal and I've learned about so many different sports. But there is one sport I would like to learn about that wasn't in the book. I am interested in this sport because...

_____

_____

_____

_____

_____

_____

_____

Illustrate your story:

Sports Study

Choose your own sport

It's research time!

Use the Internet, books, tutorials and documentaries to study this sport. Or go see a game or competition!

Draw any equipment needed for this sport.

Draw a player in uniform.

Draw a trophy or medal for this sport.

Where did this sport originate from?

_____

_____

How was this sport invented?

_____

_____

_____

Who are the main sponsors of the events for this sport?

_____

_____

What is the name of the largest competition where this sport is played? _____

_____

_____

_____

_____

Who is the #1 player of this sport? What makes them the best? How much money do they earn? Where do their earnings come from?

_____

_____

_____

_____

Would you like to play this sport? Why or why not?

_____

_____

What are the common injuries from playing this sport?

_____

_____

_____

Random fact about this sport.

_____

_____

_____

Say What?

Invent your own comic book font and add words to the picture

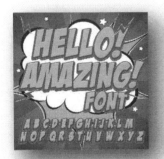
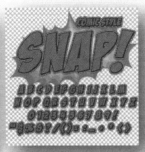
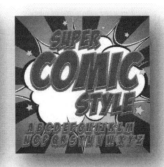
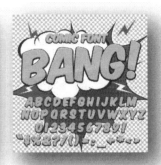

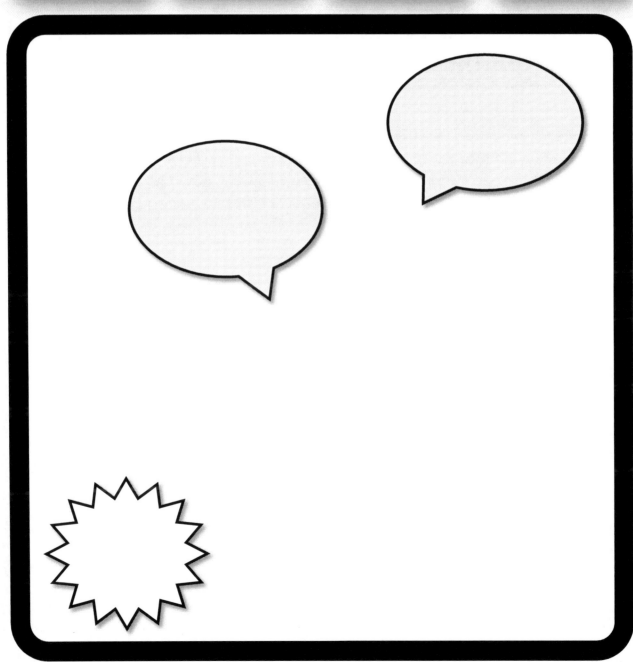

Sports News

Open a newspaper or look online!

What is happening in the world of sports today?

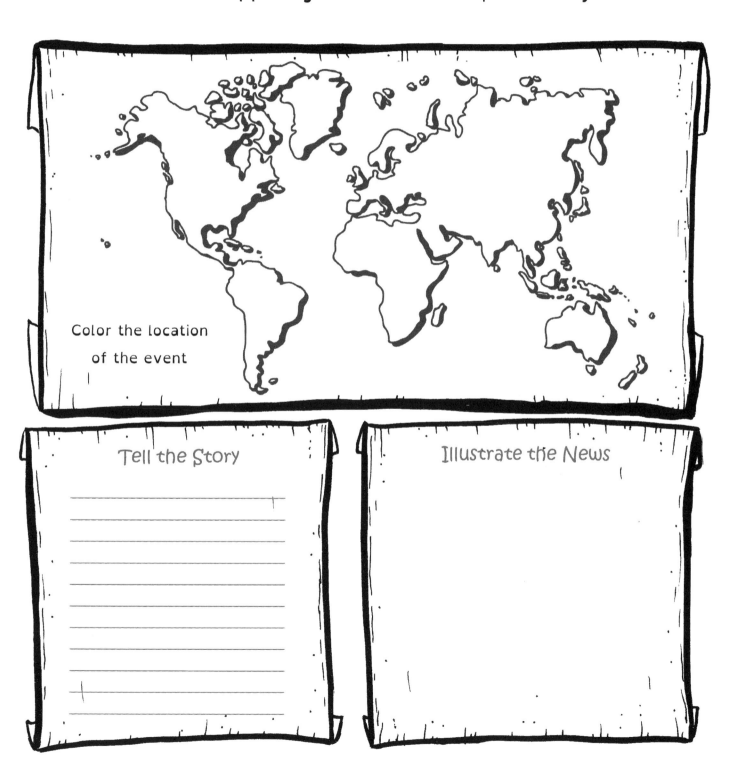

Color the location
of the event

Tell the Story

Illustrate the News

Screen Time

Watch a high-quality film, video, tutorial or sports documentary.

Title_____

Screen Time_____

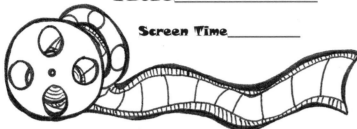

Producer_____

Actors_____

_____

_____

_____

Quotes

Draw a scene from the video.

Rating:

worst

Bad

Awful

Ok

Nice

Great

Best

Make a Comic

From the video or your imagination.

Title_____

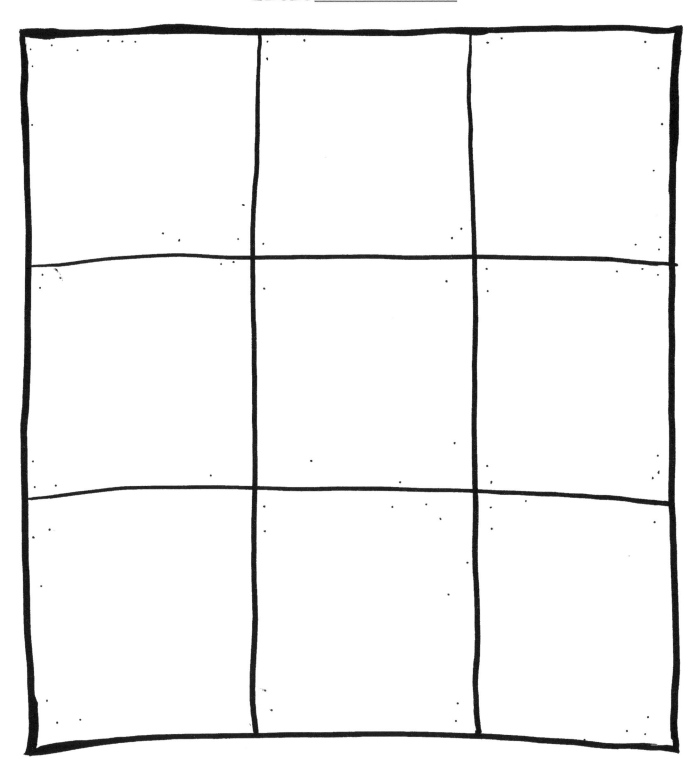

Drawing & Reading Time!

Choose a few books from your stack to focus on today.

Write down and draw anything that inspires you.

(Set a timer for 1 hour)

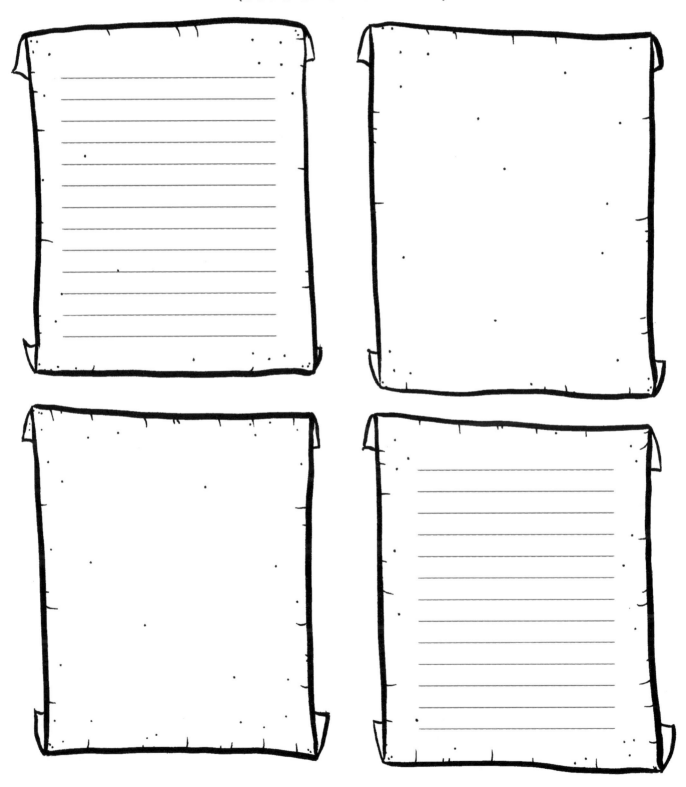

Free time!

Set the timer for 30 minutes and go outside to play, explore and practice a sport.

What do you plan to do on your free time?

What do you want to practice?

Do you have any goals?

Draw your goals!

Math Practice

Use this page for math practice,

or design a sport's field, rink or play zone

for the sport you are studying today!

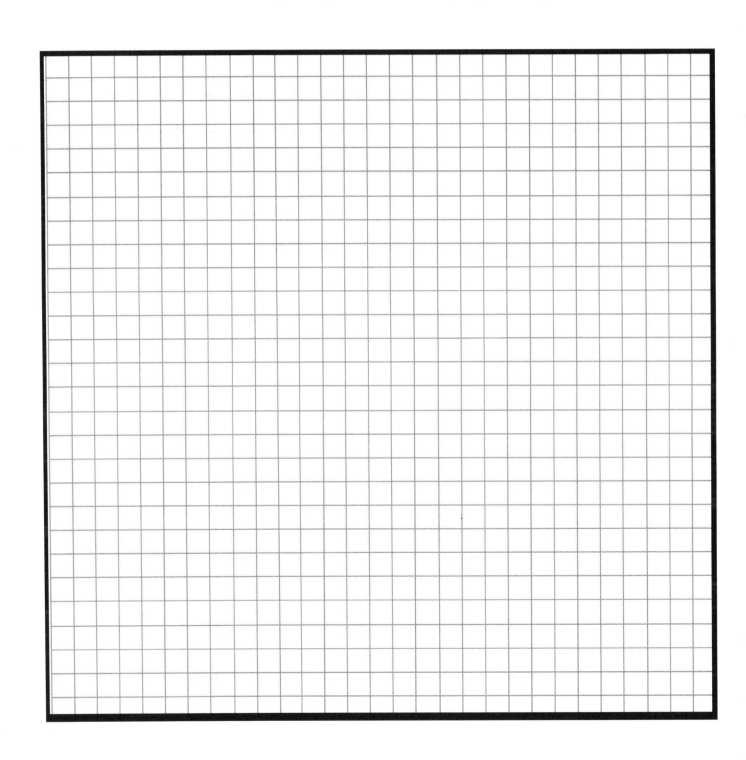

Nature Study

Take this book outside and draw anything and
everything that inspires you.

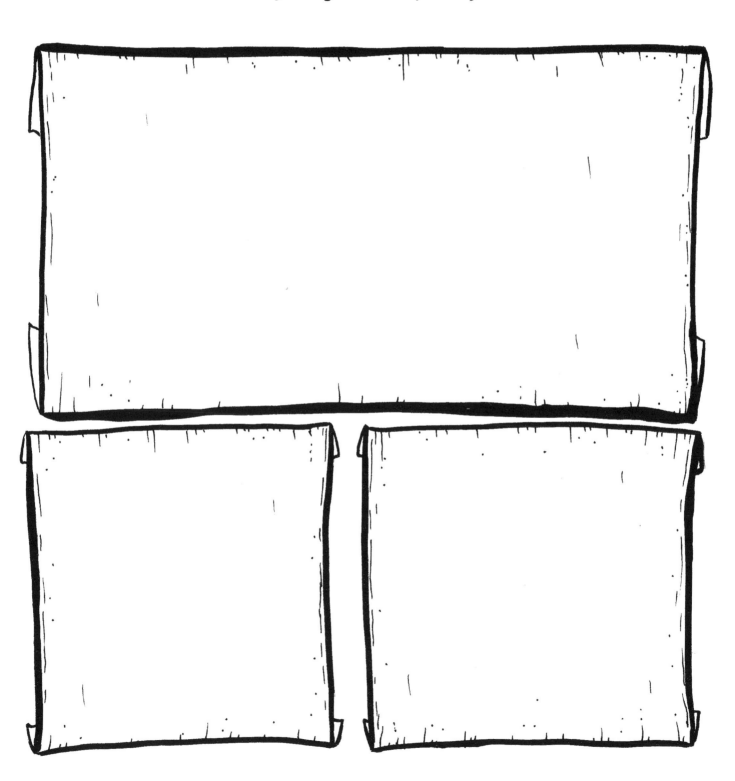

Fun-Schooling With Thinking Tree Books

Copyright Information:

Contact Us:

The Thinking Tree, LLC
+1 (USA)   317.622.8852

info@funschooling.com

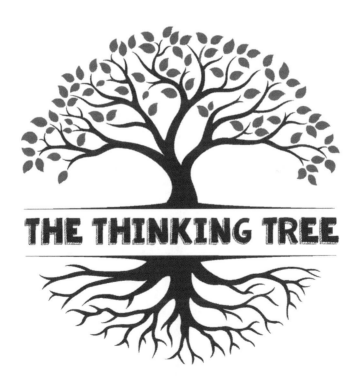

FunSchooling.com

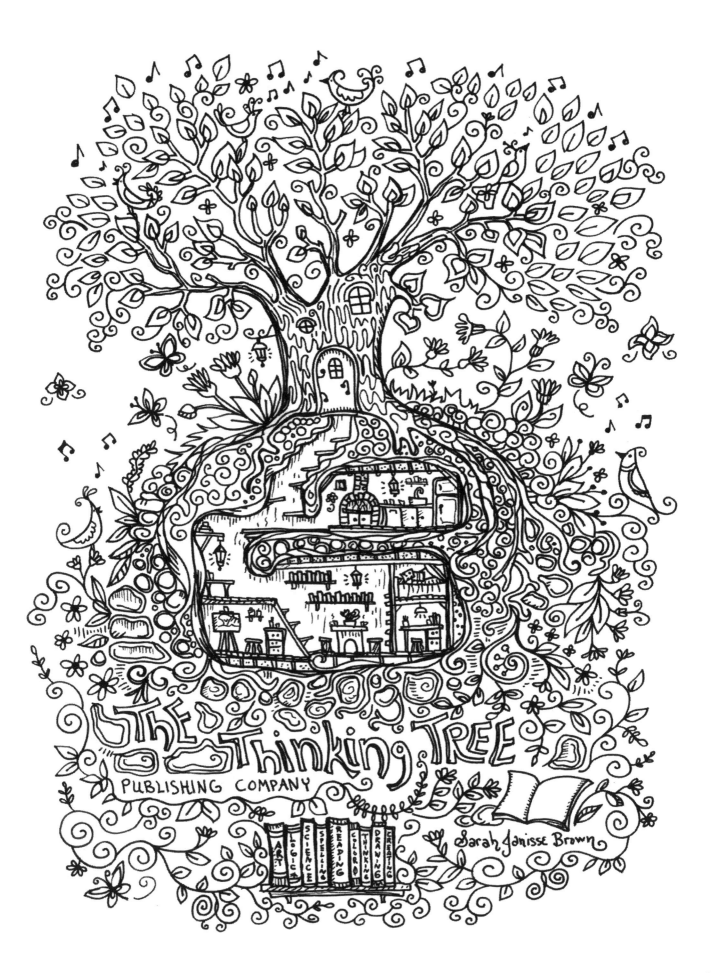

The Thinking Tree

PUBLISHING COMPANY

Sarah Janisse Brown

Made in the USA
Middletown, DE
28 July 2024

58099215R00203